Sports Nutrition

Sports Nutrition

Kary Woodruff

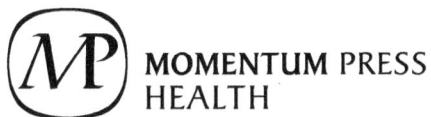

MOMENTUM PRESS
HEALTH

MOMENTUM PRESS, LLC, NEW YORK

Sports Nutrition

First published in 2016 by
Momentum Press, LLC
222 East 46th Street, New York, NY 10017
www.momentumpress.net

ISBN-13: 978-1-60650-775-9 (paperback)
ISBN-13: 978-1-60650-776-6 (e-book)

Momentum Press Nutrition and Dietetics Practice Collection

Cover and interior design by Exeter Premedia Services Private Ltd., Chennai, India

First edition: 2016

10 9 8 7 6 5 4 3 2 1

Printed in the United States of America.

This book is dedicated to my wonderfully supportive husband. I simply could not have taken on this project without your love and encouragement. Your belief in me is what inspires me to reach for great things. Thank you Eric!

Abstract

This book explores the relevance of sports nutrition for athletes and active individuals in a way that allows nutrition professionals to provide appropriate and consequential recommendations to this population. Energy, which is fundamental to the performing athlete, is defined and followed by a breakdown of energy measurement. In order to understand how energy is utilized by the working body, energy metabolism and its components are explained in a meaningful way. The concept of energy balance is introduced and is later followed up with practical recommendations for altering energy balance to assist athletes in meeting their energy and body composition goals. The macronutrients from which athletes obtain their energy—carbohydrate, protein, and fat—are described in detail, and the book includes information on food forms and metabolism. The book then offers applicable macronutrient recommendations that incorporate the timing of their intake relative to sport. There is a thorough explanation of the athlete assessment allowing the nutrition professional in gathering all relevant information to support proper meal planning and nutrient recommendations. Given the high usage of dietary supplements, this book identifies dietary supplements most commonly employed by athletes and then breaks down the quality of science behind these supplements. Finally, this book addresses special issues of concerns of athletes, such as weight management goals, potential nutrient deficiencies, and specific dietary approaches, which may need special attention when working with these individuals. The ultimate aim of this book is that a nutrition professional working with this population is armed with the information necessary to provide practical and meaningful recommendations.

Keywords

athlete assessment, body composition, carbohydrate loading, dietary supplements, eating disorders/disordered eating, energy, energy balance, energy metabolism, fluids, hydration, macronutrients—carbohydrate, protein, fat, meal planning, nutrient deficiencies such as iron deficiency, calcium, vitamin D, nutrient recommendations, race day nutrition, sports nutrition, substrate utilization, timing of intake, weight management

Contents

Preface

As a sports dietitian for many years working with athletes of all levels, sports, and backgrounds, I saw day in and day out just how crucial appropriate sports nutrition information is for athletes and active individuals. Not only does relevant sports nutrition information support optimal performance, but this material is also what helps to keep these individuals healthy while they train, and ultimately allows participation in sport to be enjoyable. Yet, time and time again, athletes would come to me with not just a lack of information, but *mis*information. That is, individuals were scouring the Internet to learn what to eat for their sport. Only a small proportion of this information is based in sound science. Individuals can be overwhelmed with trying to sort through the information. That is why they come to us—nutrition professionals—to help them understand what the science says and to apply it in a meaningful way. That is the intention of this book, to take the most current science of sports nutrition and help athletes and active individuals achieve their nutrition-related performance goals with practical recommendations. I hope you enjoy this book and find it useful in your application—whether it be personal or professional.

Acknowledgments

I would like to acknowledge the incredible work and examining eyes of my content editors: Dr. Kathie Beals, Dr. Stacie Wing Gaia, and especially the incredible attention, time, and energy of Dr. Abigail Larson. Your efforts have made this book possible. Thank you!

CHAPTER 1

Introduction to Sports Nutrition

This chapter defines sports nutrition and outlines its importance relative to performance. An overview of the scope and application of sports nutrition is also provided. The historical context, as well as an understanding of what constitutes the foundation of sports nutrition knowledge, will be addressed.

Impact of Sports Nutrition on Training and Performance

What Is Sports Nutrition?

The connection between the foods we consume and our physical capacity is indisputable. Since the time of the early Greeks and their participation in the Olympics, it has been known that our dietary habits play a significant role on our physical performance. Sports nutrition integrates the principles of exercise physiology and nutrition science in a meaningful and practical way. Exercise physiology is the understanding of the physiological, metabolic, and structural adaptations of physical activity. The body's ability to support these adaptions is mediated by the timing and intake of appropriate nutrients. Proper physical training and adequate nutrition are essential to perform to one's potential, and having one without the other will result in suboptimal performance. All aspects of movement, muscular strength, agility, endurance, flexibility, and coordination require a complex interaction of energy and nutrients. Understanding the principles of how energy is transferred from the foods we eat into the movements we make is required for useful application of sport nutrition knowledge.

Science has long supported the significance of appropriate nutrition strategies for fueling activity and achieving optimal performance. A classic research study by Costill et al. (1971) illustrates what happens when appropriate nutrient recommendations are not followed. In this study five endurance runners ran 16.1 km (10 miles) at a relatively high intensity on three successive days. These athletes consumed a normal, mixed diet that fell below the recommended carbohydrate intake for their sport. Muscle biopsies revealed that prolonged, intense exercise on successive days resulted in a continued decline in resting muscle glycogen stores. This study demonstrates that athletes who train hard on consecutive days and do not refuel with adequate carbohydrate may experience impaired performance on consequent days.

In working with athletes, providing real-life scenarios can elucidate some of these concepts. For example, the importance of sports nutrition can be demonstrated with the following analogy. Imagine a set of identical twins. In addition to having the same genetic makeup, these twins have indistinguishable technical skills, cardiovascular conditioning and endurance, and equal strength. Everything about their athletic capacity is identical. Yet, if one of these athletes is fueling better, that is, giving their bodies the proper types and amounts of nutrients in the appropriate timing, this athlete will outperform their counterpart. Sports nutrition makes a significant difference in one's performance and physical ability and can ultimately give an athlete the competitive edge over their opponents.

Sports nutrition has a wide range of applications and utility. From the weekend warrior to the highly trained competitive athlete, fueling appropriately helps individuals achieve their fitness and performance goals. Sound nutrition strategies support recreational athletes in increasing fitness levels, including cardiovascular fitness and strength gains. Appropriate fueling strategies can help daily exercise to be more enjoyable and also supports mood and cognitive function. Sufficient macronutrients (carbohydrates, proteins, and fats) are especially important for athletes, as they are essential to fuel their training, and both macro- and micronutrients, including vitamins and minerals, are needed for recovery, repair, and growth. Nutrition also plays a significant role in achieving and maintaining good health status, as immune function relies upon good nutrition practices. Athletes seeking weight management goals will rely upon appropriate dietary practices to safely meet their objectives without compromising health or performance. Sound nutrition principles are the cornerstone of a healthy foundation for activities of daily living all the way to elite athletic training.

Sports Nutrition: Research and Practitioners

While the science of sports nutrition has undergone tremendous growth in the past few decades, the understanding that the food we eat impacts our physical performance has long been understood. Even Greek athletes in ancient Roman times abided by a set of beliefs in which certain nutrition habits were thought to optimize their training. Though the specifics of what the athlete's diet looked like were constantly changing, not much has changed in 2,000 years! As far back as the third century BC, athletes were studying how diet impacted performance (Grivetti and Applegate 1997); however, it has only been in the past several decades that the field of sports nutrition has seen significant growth. It has transitioned from a generalized, imprecise body of knowledge filled with myths and misconceptions, to a specialized, robust science with a strong body of research to support sound recommendations to athletes of all levels, skills, and types of sports. Yet, more than just a science, sports nutrition is an art form. A sport dietitian—an expert practitioner of sports nutrition—takes research-based findings and applies them in an individualized manner. The sport dietitian looks at the whole picture of the athlete with whom they are working, considering their sport type and the demands of the sport, the goals of the athlete, and the training and competitive level at which the athlete is performing, and customizes these science-based recommendations. It is an art as much as it is a science.

The principles of sports nutrition are derived from research conducted with scientific rigor. This includes research from well-designed studies published in peer-reviewed journals free from subjective bias. The evidence-based recommendations used by sports dietitians do not stem from the results of a single research study, rather these recommendations are a synthesis of results from multiple studies examining the same topic. Yet, where do most Americans obtain their nutrition knowledge? In one survey of over 1,000 Americans that asked which resources they utilized to eat healthier, the majority of individuals reported using friends and family (32 percent), followed by using a weight loss plan (22 percent), and apps or other websites (22 percent) (International Food Information Council Foundation 2015). Only 6 percent of individuals reported relying upon a Registered Dietitian Nutritionist for credible information. In a study specific to athletes (runners), the main sources of sports nutrition information were friends (57 percent), magazines (45 percent), and websites (32 percent) (Flynn 2014). Again (sports) dietitians or other credible nutrition professionals were not utilized as primary resources for credible nutrition information. Anyone can conduct an Internet search on the optimal diet for an athlete, yet the resulting information may or may not be accurate. Some of this information may mislead athletes to adopt fad diets, consume potentially dangerous dietary supplements, or other unhealthy dietary practices.

Individuals looking for sports nutrition information need to be sure to obtain their information from credible sources. One challenge for consumers is that there is a lack of understanding of *who is* an expert in sports nutrition. Sports nutrition textbooks, professional websites (such as scandpg.org—the sports nutrition practice group of the Academy of Nutrition and Dietetics), and **Certified Specialist in Sports Dietetics** (CSSD) are all considered expert sources for sport nutrition information. An individual with the CSSD certification is not only a Registered Dietitian Nutritionist, but someone who has practiced for a minimum of 2 years working with athletes and active individuals, and has taken a certifying examination specific to sports nutrition. Other fitness professionals including certified Athletic Trainers (ATC) and personal trainers may have received some sports nutrition information, but their scope will be more limited than a CSSD. Helping to provide sports nutrition education as well as directing consumers to other credible sources is essential not just for optimal nutrition and performance, but also potentially for the safety of the athlete, as information garnered from noncredible sources can result in unsafe nutrition and supplementation practices.

Overview of the Book

This book will dissect the fundamentals of sports nutrition and provide research-based recommendations for their application. A thorough explanation of the term energy, as it relates to food and physical activity, as well as how it is measured will be offered. The role of each macronutrient (carbohydrate, protein, and fat) will be examined within the context of physical activity and energy metabolism. Recommendations for the amount and timing of each macronutrient will be discussed, as will appropriate food sources. Hydration will be addressed and will include current controversies over best hydration practices. Dietary supplements is another hot topic in sports nutrition, and this book will help the reader assess the efficacy of some of the most popular supplements based upon scientific evidence.

This text will apply the principles and recommendations from previous chapters through the process of assessing the nutrient needs of individual athletes. Specific components of an athlete's diet will be addressed, including competition diet, concerns regarding weight loss or weight gain, and identifying specific nutrient deficiencies. Finally, the bigger picture of an athlete's diet and essential components to planning an athlete's diet will be acknowledged.

Definition

Certified Specialist in Sports Dietetics (CSSD)—a Registered Dietitian nutritionist who is an expert in the application of sports nutrition. These individuals have successfully completed the board examination, following 2 years working as a Registered Dietitian with a minimum of 1,500 hours of sports nutrition practice.

References

Costill, D.L., R. Bowers, G. Branam, and K. Sparks. 1971. "Muscle Glycogen Utilization During Prolonged Exercise on Successive Days." *Journal of Applied Physiology* 31, no. 6, pp. 834–38.

Flynn, L. 2014. *Marathon Runners and Their Nutrition Views, Practices, and Sources of Nutrition Information* [Theses – ALL] Paper 47. Syracuse University.

Grivetti, L.E., and E.A. Applegate. 1997. "From Olympia to Atlanta: A Cultural-Historical Perspective on Diet and Athletic Training." *The Journal of Nutrition* 127, no. 5, pp. 860S–68S.

International Food Information Council Foundation. 2015. "Food & Health Survey 2015." www.foodinsight.org/sites/default/files/2015-Food-and-Health-Survey-Full-Report.pdf (accessed August 10, 2015).

CHAPTER 2

Measurement of Energy

All food consumed in the diet is digested, metabolized, and then absorbed through various enzymatic and physiological processes. The resulting metabolites are then used to meet immediate energy needs or are stored for later use depending upon the nutritional and physiological state of the body. All processes of the body require energy. Energy is the capacity to do work, and without energy we would not be able to sustain life, let alone participate in competitive sport. Understanding basic principles of energy transfer and measurement is essential for understanding the sports nutrition recommendations and applications.

This chapter examines direct and indirect methods used to quantify energy intake and expenditure. Energy intake refers to the energy content of food and beverages consumed, and energy expenditure refers to the energy utilized by the body. Energy balance can be calculated by subtracting energy that is expended from energy consumed.

Energy intake is a relatively easy concept to grasp (total energy of all foods and beverages consumed). Energy expenditure is somewhat more abstract and has three components including resting energy expenditure (REE), thermic effect of food (TEF), and energy expended through physical activity (PA). Sports nutrition professionals can measure energy expenditure using direct and indirect measures. The measurement method selected varies in terms of accuracy and validity, and the choice of the assessment tool is most often based on practical and logistical considerations. The fundamentals of energy balance and measurement of energy are essential to understanding how energy is utilized by athletes and allows the sports dietitian to make appropriate energy recommendations.

Measuring Energy

Unit of Measurement

From the act of stretching first thing in the morning, to running a marathon, all bodily movements require **energy**. Energy is what fuels activity and exercise and comes from the calories that individuals consume; both quality and quantity of calories impact the energy available for sport. While the idea of energy may seem simple, actually measuring energy can be quite complex. As with any measurement, the appropriate unit must be identified. The International System of Units (SI units) has been developed by the scientific community as a set of standardized weights and measures that utilize the metric system. SI units establish the official units of energy used among most research communities globally, though this chapter also identifies units commonly used in the United States.

The SI unit of measurement for mechanical energy is the **joule**. Energy can also be understood and measured in terms of heat, which better represents how energy is transformed in living systems. A calorie (lowercase c) may be a familiar unit of measurement. It represents the amount of heat needed to raise the temperature of one gram of water by 1°C. Because this amount of heat is so small in relation to the amount of energy measured in food or expended during activity, using Calorie (uppercase C) or kilocalorie (kcal) is more practical. A Calorie, or kcal, equals 1,000 calories and is the amount of heat needed to increase the temperature of 1 kg (or 1 L) of water by 1°C. In practical terms, Calories, or kcal, is a measurement of the energy content of a food or liquid; kcal can also be used to determine the specific energy requirements of an activity. Scientific research still relies upon SI units (joules in the case of energy), so the following conversions may be helpful to know:

- 1 calorie = 4.184 joules
- 1 kcal = 1,000 calories
- 1 kcal = 4,184 joules, *or,*
- 1 kcal = 4.184 kilojoules

Throughout this text, kcal and calories will be used interchangeably, however, both reference 1,000 calories (lowercase c).

Measuring Energy in Food

Humans obtain energy from foods and beverages. Measuring the exact caloric, or energy, value of food can be achieved through direct calorimetry. In this method, a food sample is burned in a bomb calorimeter that measures the heat produced by measuring the change in temperature in the chamber. The heat is directly measured; therefore, this is considered a direct measure. The three macronutrients, carbohydrate, protein, and fat, have all been analyzed for their energy content using direct calorimetry, as have many combinations of macronutrients in common foods. In the late 1890s and early 1900s, W.O. Atwater and colleagues developed the Atwater general factor system, which was later modified in the 1950s to the Atwater specific factor system. Both Atwater factor systems provide estimates of metabolizable energy (ME), or the amount of energy that remains available to the body after accounting for losses attributable to incomplete digestion of food resulting in fecal and urinary losses, and small amounts lost from the body surface. Carbohydrate and protein have an energy or kcal value of 4.2 kcal/g, alcohol has 7.0 kcal/g, and fat has 9.4 kcal/g. Using the precise kilocalorie value for each macronutrient makes for tedious calculations, so they are rounded to the nearest whole number.

- Carbohydrates = 4 kcal/g
- Protein = 4 kcal/g
- Alcohol = 7 kcal/g
- Fat = 9 kcal/g

Since these values are rounded, when they are multiplied by several factors, such as in the case of determining the caloric value of a meal, this could result in under- or overestimation of total calorie content. Food labels should also be viewed as estimates because, although the most accurate calorie value of a food would be measured via direct calorimetry, this is rarely the case. Few packaged and processed foods have been measured directly for their caloric content for many reasons, including cost of direct calorimetry, needed equipment, time constraints, and the impracticality of burning every manufactured food item. Instead, food processing software with comprehensive databases is used as a proxy to estimate the calorie value. This is considered an indirect measure because the actual food item is not being measured.

Even if direct calorimetry was used to measure every food product available, only the heat produced from food samples is being measured. Direct (or indirect) calorimetry cannot measure the amount of energy that is actually transferred to the body through the process of digestion, metabolism, and absorption; this amount cannot be directly measured. Given these limitations, calories should only be viewed as estimates. "Calorie counting" as a method to change body composition may result in over- or underestimation of actual caloric intake. People who try and count every calorie that they consume must realize they are only estimating their energy intake and are not getting an exact measurement. For example, packaged food items are allowed to be 10 percent higher or lower in kcal content than the value indicated on the nutrition facts; so even if you were able to count every calorie consumed, you may have over- or underestimated your caloric intake by more than 10 percent.

Measuring Energy Expenditure

Just as getting a precise value for energy intake in individuals is quite challenging, measuring human energy expenditure is neither an exact nor a straightforward process. Direct and indirect energy expenditure methods are described as follows.

Direct Calorimetry

Direct calorimetry measures energy expenditure in humans based on the same principles that measure the calorie content of food. That is, the heat an individual produces is proportional to the energy one is expending. A bomb calorimeter, which, in this case is an enclosed chamber large enough to hold an individual, has specialized sensors that measure the change in temperature when the individual is engaging in activity. This change in temperature measures the heat being produced and thus assesses the amount of energy being expended. Because of the advanced technology and equipment required, direct calorimetry is an expensive assessment and not without limitations. Exercise machines housed within the chamber may produce their own heat during use, resulting in an over-estimation of heat produced by the exercising individual.

Further, not all heat produced from the body is "liberated" and thus may not be measured; rather, in the process known as excess postexercise oxygen consumption (EPOC), the body expends additional energy in efforts to restore homeostasis. Processes of EPOC include replenishing the energy resources, such as phosphocreatine and muscle glycogen, utilized during exercise; reoxygenating blood and restoring hormonal balance; and resuming normal ventilation and heart rate. EPOC also includes expending energy to restore normalcy of the body temperature that was elevated due to the metabolic heat produced from working muscle. The result is that not all heat is "liberated" during exercise but continues to be released after exercise is completed. Thus, detection of heat changes during exercise will fail to capture all of the heat produced in that time. These limitations must be taken into consideration when interpreting energy expenditure results; however, in comparison to other measures of energy expenditure, direct calorimetry is the most accurate method and is still utilized in research settings.

Indirect Measures

The equipment and technology required for direct calorimetry do not make it a feasible measurement of energy expenditure for most practical applications. The small enclosed chamber is also not very representative of the environment in which "real-life" athletes perform and thus limits the types of activities that can be measured. Thus, more practical methods have been developed and are more commonly used to measure energy expended during physical activity and exercise.

Indirect calorimetry. Indirect calorimetry is based on the assumption that heat produced during activity can be assessed by measuring the volume of oxygen (O_2) consumed (VO_2) and carbon dioxide (CO_2) expired. As energy expenditure increases, the amount of oxygen consumed and carbon dioxide expired increase proportionately. Indirect calorimetry thus allows for the calculation of the respiratory quotient, or RQ. The RQ measures the ratio of the volume of carbon dioxide (V_c) produced to the volume of oxygen (V_o) consumed:

$$RQ = V_c/V_o$$

Volumes of O_2 consumed and CO_2 produced depend upon which fuel source is being metabolized by the individual. An RQ of 1.0 indicates that the individual is metabolizing pure carbohydrate; an RQ of 0.7 represents pure fat oxidation. Values in between represent oxidation of carbohydrate and fat and depend upon the exact number to estimate the contribution of each macronutrient. This measurement of O_2 and CO_2 gas exchange also allows the calculation of energy expenditure indirectly and thus is a measure of indirect calorimetry since the RQ value corresponds to a caloric value for each liter of CO_2 produced. This technology also has the capacity to measure maximal oxygen consumption, or VO_2 max. VO_2 max is the maximal rate of oxygen consumed during incremental exercise, measured as mL/kg/min and is often used as a measurement of aerobic capacity. Application of VO_2 max will be discussed later in this chapter.

VO_2 can be measured in liters per minute (L/min), or as an adjusted measurement relative to body weight, as milliliters of oxygen consumed per kilogram of body weight per minute (mL/kg/min). One liter of oxygen consumed approximates 5 kcal of energy expended, and total oxygen consumption of a given activity can be used to calculate energy expenditure (total liters consumed × 5 kcal). Energy expenditure of a given activity is typically expressed in terms of kilocalories expended per minute (expressed as kcal/min). It is important to understand this is a measurement of total kilocalories expended during the time frame and not just the kilocalories used for the specific activity, because the measurement includes calories expended for other metabolic functions. Thus, when athletes see their caloric expenditure for specific activities based on indirect calorimetry, this is total energy expended for all physiological processes during that time and not just the calories used for the activity.

Indirect calorimetry can be performed in the same calorimetry chambers used for direct calorimetry, since these sealed chambers are an optimal environment in which to measure gas exchange. For practical considerations, however, the most common form of indirect calorimetry is an open-circuit spirometry system in which a computerized mobile cart, or metabolic cart, allows the individual to breathe ambient air. The cart has technology that measures the amount of air inhaled, analyzes the oxygen and carbon dioxide content in the air, and measures the amount of carbon dioxide expired from the individual.

The portability of this system and lack of requirement for a sealed chamber permit the measurement of energy expenditure in educational settings. Semiportable metabolic carts can be used to measure energy expenditure in exercise physiology labs. These semiportable metabolic carts require access to a laboratory with equipment that is fairly expensive, which limits the practicality of these systems. Given that the individual is physically connected to the cart via a tube, there are only limited activities that can be measured, such as running, cycling, and rowing on treadmills and ergometers. Many other sports and activities cannot be measured using this technology, limiting its application.

In order to assess energy expenditure in an athlete's actual environment and not in a research laboratory, more portable metabolic systems have been developed. These portable carts can be used in sport-specific contexts. A trade-off is that their accuracy is not as high as the laboratory measurement systems, though they still provide an acceptable measurement of energy expenditure with good reliability (Vogler, Rice, and Gore 2010). While these portable metabolic carts cannot be used in all sport contexts, the technology is continually evolving, helping to broaden their applicability to athletes.

Portable metabolic carts have application not only to athletes but also in clinical settings. Indirect calorimetry using metabolic measurement systems is one of the most accurate assessments of resting energy expenditure (REE). **REE**, or **resting metabolic rate** (RMR), provides an estimate of the calories an individual needs at rest and can be measured by indirect calorimetry. Individuals lay in the supine position and breathe into a face mask attached to the metabolic cart for a period of time, typically about 20 to 30 minutes, and up to several hours for increased accuracy. Individuals should not eat for several hours or exercise for at least 24 hours before having REE or RMR measured. Measurements are most accurate when conducted early in the morning and when the individual has been resting quietly for a designated amount of time (such as 20 minutes).

To obtain a more precise assessment of basal metabolic needs, basal energy expenditure (BEE) or **basal metabolic rate** (BMR) can be measured. This is the amount of energy expended at complete rest. Individuals spend the night in a research laboratory so that their measurement can be taken immediately upon waking and before rising. Because this protocol is not always feasible or accessible, RMR is more often measured in practical settings such as health clinics and sports medicine facilities. For both BMR or RMR assessments, the individual should have refrained from strenuous exercise within the past 24 hours and should not have eaten in the past several hours (or be at least 8 hours fasted in the case of BMR), and the assessment should be conducted in a temperature-controlled environment that is free from loud or distracting noises. These protocols prevent external factors from affecting an individual's RMR or BMR.

Indirect calorimetry is often considered a gold standard method for assessing REE. There is good accuracy and reliability when the procedure is completed with calibrated equipment (Pinheiro Volp et al. 2011). Metabolic carts can also measure VO_2 max, which can be a useful training tool for athletes. While there is greater portability in newer technology, the trade-off is that a greater margin of error is introduced (Vogler, Rice, and Gore 2010). Additionally, the technology can be quite expensive and requires the presence of a trained administrator.

Indirect calorimetry can measure RMR and energy expended during physical activity; yet, in order to understand how these measurements fit into the overall energy needs of an athlete, one must understand the basic principles of energy balance.

Energy Balance

Understanding how energy intake and energy expenditure interact and affect overall energy balance is essential in order to provide appropriate energy recommendations for meeting nutrition and performance goals. Energy balance is achieved when calories consumed through food and liquids are equal to the calories expended by the body to maintain basic physiological processes and perform physical work. Figure 2.1 illustrates this concept by using a balanced scale as a visual aid.

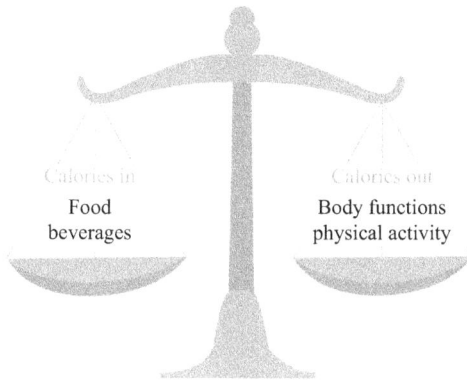

Figure 2.1 Energy balance

Measuring the energy content of the food and beverages humans consume is sometimes termed the "input" side of the energy balance equation. The "output" is the energy humans expend on all metabolic processes as well as any form of activity, including activities of daily living (ADLs) and structured exercise. Athletes must have a thorough understanding of how energy balance affects body weight and performance. If an athlete's inputs, that is, energy from food and beverages, equals the energy one expends (the outputs) on a daily basis, their weight will stay the same. If the input side of the equation is greater than the output side, then an athlete will experience weight gain. This may enhance performance if the weight gain comes from lean body mass (LBM), or may negatively impact performance if the weight is in the form of fat mass (FM). An athlete whose inputs are less than the outputs will likely lose weight. Depending upon the type of weight that is lost and the rate of weight loss, this may enhance performance if body fat is lost at an appropriate rate as with an endurance athlete who has less body mass to carry, or may impair performance in the case of an athlete whose rapid weight loss results in loss of LBM and inadequate energy. Energy balance is very consequential for weight management and performance.

Understanding energy balance is crucial for the sports nutrition practitioner working with an athlete who has weight management goals. Some athletes wish to maintain their weight (input equals the output) and thus should be in energy balance. Some athletes want to gain weight in the form of LBM, and in this case inputs need to be greater than the outputs to be in positive energy balance. Athletes wanting to lose weight need to ensure the inputs are less than the outputs and thus need to be in negative energy balance. This is not as simple and straightforward as it may seem. To support athletes in these goals, the sports nutrition professional first needs to measure both sides of the equation before any recommendations can be made.

Measuring Energy Input

Measuring the energy content in food has been described earlier and is relatively straightforward. The most accurate form of measurement is a bomb calorimeter, though most often calorie values found on food labels are derived from food processing software. Actually tracking the foods an individual consumes in order to determine total energy intake is a little more complex. Most often, daily intake is estimated using dietary records, or food logs. These require an individual to track one's food and beverage intake and amount for 1 to 7 days. These paper or electronic logs can then be analyzed using computer software that calculates the energy value of the foods and beverages consumed. Alternatively, smartphone apps allow individuals to record their daily intake throughout the day, and this technology then computes the nutrient analysis without requiring additional software. Regardless of the analysis method, the recorded information must be very detailed to be accurate. A significant and common source of error when estimating energy intake is the underreporting of portion sizes and omission of beverages. Causes of underreporting and omission include poor memory or recall if food is not recorded at the time of consumption, failure to measure portion sizes, and possible self-consciousness over one's food choices. All of these result in the underestimation of total energy intake. Regardless, food records are still the most practical method available for estimating energy intake. Athlete assessment will go into further detail regarding use of food records (see Chapter 5).

Measuring Energy Output

Because the output side of the equation, energy expenditure, has different components, this assessment is more complex. Total energy expenditure (TEE), sometimes known as total daily energy expenditure (TDEE), is the amount of energy used by the body in 24 hours. TEE has three components: REE comprising 60 to 75 percent of TEE, the TEF comprising 10 percent of TEE, and PA comprising 20 to 30 percent (see Figure 2.2).

Resting Energy Expenditure

REE or RMR is the amount of energy used by the body in a wakeful state while resting. If one were to lie in bed for a 24-hour period that included periods of wakefulness, REE would be the total amount of energy they would expend. Components of REE include blood circulation throughout the body, respiration, body temperature regulation, central nervous system functioning, and other physiological functions. Liver, brain, heart, and kidney tissues use up most of the REE since these are the most metabolically active tissues. Because REE, or RMR, measures energy expenditure in a wakeful and alert state, REE is about 10 percent higher than BEE, or BMR.

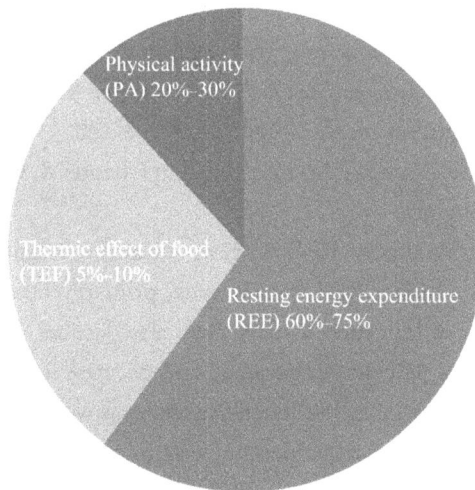

Figure 2.2 Components of TEE

REE comprises 60 to 75 percent of TEE, though the actual amount varies within and between individuals. Body composition, body mass, sex, age, height, genetics, hormonal factors, nutritional status, environmental conditions, cigarette, and caffeine use all effect REE. REE can vary within an individual from day to day based on the demands placed upon the body. Some individuals may wish to increase REE to help with weight loss efforts, and while some determinants of REE cannot be altered, there are some modifiable factors. Body composition is one modifiable determinant of RMR. Individuals with greater LBM will have a higher REE because LBM is more metabolically active than FM. That is, LBM uses more energy even when at rest. In fact, even at rest, muscle tissue requires about three times as many calories as fat tissue.

Nutritional status has the potential to alter REE as well. When energy intake is drastically reduced, in efforts to lose weight or during times of illness, the body responds by going into a state of **adaptive thermogenesis**, commonly known as starvation mode. This process is an evolutionary adaptation by the body to become more efficient with what energy it receives by depressing metabolic rate. The function of this metabolic efficiency is to attempt to attenuate the loss of muscle and FM. Since the body does not know how long the starvation period will last, this response happens quickly. Historically, during periods of famine, energy efficiency was advantageous for survival; however, for the individual looking to lose weight, decreased metabolic rate works against weight loss efforts. In fact, severe caloric restriction has been shown to lower RMR by as much as 18 to 25 percent (Onur et al. 2005; Russell et al. 2001). Depressed metabolic rate will be discussed in more detail in Chapter 8, which addresses weight management.

Some determinants of REE, such as sex and age, cannot be modified. Men have a higher REE than women, primarily because men have a larger amount of lean muscle mass. REE also declines as an individual ages (about 1 to 2 percent per decade). This decrease is partly a result of loss of muscle mass due to lower activity levels, as well as recent research indicating there is an age-dependent increase in markers related to muscle protein breakdown (Tanner et al. 2015). This decline can be mitigated by engaging in resistance exercise throughout the life cycle. Other factors that are somewhat modifiable, although not always practical, such as colder temperatures, higher altitudes, caffeine intake, and smoking, can temporarily increase REE, though their effect is minimal and does not have a lasting effect.

Measuring Resting Energy Expenditure. Indirect calorimetry. As previously described, measuring REE using indirect calorimetry can provide a reasonably accurate measurement if the correct procedures are followed; however, this method is not always feasible due to either the expenses or access, or both, to the necessary technology. In these cases, other estimates, such as predictive equations, can be used to estimate REE.

Predictive equations. In the absence of an indirect calorimeter, predictive equations can be used to estimate REE. Various characteristics of individuals, including weight, height, sex, age, are included in an equation used to calculate an estimated REE. Predictive equations must be considered a loose estimate because only a few selected factors that affect REE are accounted for. Furthermore, these equations are population specific; that is, they will be most valid when used within the population from which they have been validated. Measurement accuracy will decrease when a specific equation is used on an individual from a different population. Unfortunately, there are insufficient research studies to provide valid equations for all existing populations.

For the general public, there are many equations available to estimate REE. The four most common are the Mifflin–St. Jeor equation, the Harris–Benedict equation, the Owen equation, and the World Health Organization/Food and Agriculture Organization/United Nations University (WHO/FAO/UNU) equations (see Table 2.1). In a study that compared these four equations to a criterion measurement, a hand-held metabolic calorimeter, it was shown that the Harris–Benedict equation best predicted REE across all BMI groups, and that the Mifflin–St. Jeor equation best predicted REE among obese populations (Hasson et al. 2011). However, these equations may be less accurate when applied to athletes because they do not take body composition into consideration. Specifically, fat free mass (FFM) including muscle tissue is more metabolically active than FM and increases REE (Hall et al. 2012). It is assumed that athletes have a greater percentage of FFM at a given weight, and thus it is expected that they would have a higher REE compared to an individual of the same weight but with less FFM. In fact, research has shown that the amount of FFM an individual has is one of the major determinants of REE regardless of body weight and size (Oshima et al. 2011; Taguchi et al. 2011). Given the importance of FFM as it relates to REE, it is recommended the Cunningham equation be used with athletes because of its inclusion of this component (see Table 2.1). In order to use the Cunningham equation, the amount of FFM must be known. This can be achieved with body composition assessments such as underwater weighing and air displacement plethysmography (the BodPod). These and other body composition assessments will be discussed in Chapter 5.

Table 2.1 Predictive equations

Predictive equations for estimating RMR
Harris–Benedict equation:
Males: RMR (kcal/day) = 66.5 + 13.75 × wt (kg) + 5 × ht (cm) − 6.76 × age (years)
Females: RMR (kcal/day) = 655 + 9.56 × wt (kg) + 1.7 × ht (cm) − 4.7 × age (years)
Mifflin–St. Jeor equation:
Males: RMR (kcal/day) = (9.99 × wt) + (6.25 × ht) − (4.92 × age) + 5
Females: RMR (kcal/day) = (9.99 × wt) + (6.25 × ht) − (4.92 × age) − 161
Note: weight (wt) is in kg; height (ht) is in cm; age is in years
Owen equation:
Males: RMR (kcal/day) = 10.2 × wt (kg) + 875
Females: RMR (kcal/day) = 7.18 × wt (kg) + 620
WHO/FAO/UNU equation:
Age (years):
Males: 18–30: RMR (kcal/day) = 15.3 × wt (kg) − 27 × ht (m) + 717
31–60: RMR (kcal/day) = 11.3 × wt (kg) + 16 × ht (m) + 901
> 60: RMR (kcal/day) = 8.8 × wt (kg) + 1,129 × ht (m) − 1,071
Females: 18–30: RMR (kcal/day) = 13.3 × wt (kg) + 334 × ht (m) + 35
31–60: RMR (kcal/day) = 8.7 wt (kg) − 25 × ht (m) + 865
> 60: RMR (kcal/day) = 9.2 × wt (kg) + 637 × ht (m) − 302
Cunningham equation:
Kcal/day = 500 + 22 × FFM (kg) (Cunningham 1980)

Note: The Harris–Benedict equation, Mifflin–St. Jeor equation, Owen equation, and WHO/FAO/UNU are four equations that can be used to estimate RMR.

While indirect calorimetry produces the most accurate measurements of REE, technology and expense can limit an athlete's access to this method. Instead, predictive equations can be used. These calculations are less accurate but may be more practical in some sports nutrition settings. Many equations are available; however, due to its inclusion of FFM, using the Cunningham is preferred within an athletic population.

Thermic Effect of Food

The TEF, also known as dietary-induced thermogenesis, is the amount of energy expended for digestion, absorption, metabolism, and storage of food in the body. This amount is above REE and comprises about 10 percent of TEE. The TEF is affected by various characteristics of the food consumed, though the total energy (calorie) content of the food has the greatest impact on TEF. The macronutrient content of the food (carbohydrate, protein, fat, and alcohol) also impacts the TEF. Fat has the lowest TEF using only 2 to 3 percent of the calories consumed from fat. Carbohydrate has a TEF of 5 to 10 percent of carbohydrate calories consumed, and protein has the highest TEF, requiring 20 to 30 percent of calories ingested from protein for its metabolism that relates to protein's impact of satiety after a meal. This is one of the reasons why diets high in protein are reported to have greater satiety and may help with weight management goals. While alcohol has a TEF of about 10 to 30 percent, it does not seem to have the same effect on satiety as protein (Westerterp 2004).

Measuring Thermic Effect of Food.   TEF can be measured in a research laboratory. This is rarely done because it is usually not feasible nor is it very practical. Instead, TEF can be calculated by multiplying 10 percent to the total caloric intake of the diet. For example, an individual consuming 2,400 calories would have a TEF of 240 calories. However, because the contribution of TEF is relatively small compared to that of RMR, it usually is not factored into TEE estimates. TEF lasts only 1 to 2 hours after consuming a mixed meal and so the overall impact is fairly minimal.

Physical Activity

Physical activity, or PA, is the third component of TEE. This includes the amount of energy expended on ADLs, or the basic tasks of everyday life. Cooking, cleaning, getting dressed, energy expended while working, at school, and other daily tasks are all considered ADLs. Physical activity expenditure also includes the energy used for structured exercise; for athletes, this amount can be quite considerable.

Physical activity energy expenditure is the most variable component of TEE. Physical activity is estimated to comprise about 20 to 30 percent of TEE, though this value can vary widely according to the lifestyle habits and exercise patterns of the individual. Individuals have the most control over this component of TEE; minimal changes can be made to REE, and TEF is relatively static. Yet, the amount of energy one expends on a daily basis engaging in activity can have a profound effect on total energy expended. If an individual has a sedentary job where one sits most of the day, and does not engage in structured exercise or in other daily activities such as cleaning or gardening, the PA energy expenditure will be relatively minor. On the other hand, individuals working active jobs, such as manual labor positions, and also exercise on a daily basis will have a significantly greater contribution of PA energy expenditure toward TEE.

Even within an individual, daily activity can vary greatly. An athlete who works a sedentary job and has a "rest" day from training may only have a small PA expenditure. A 120 lb female runner, for example, who works a desk job and does not exercise on a given day, may only need 1,750 calories to meet her energy needs. This represents a 20 percent increase in calories over her RMR. On a hard training day where she has a long run and then engages in house cleaning the rest of the day may need upward of 2,600 calories. This is an almost 90 percent increase in calories over her RMR! Obviously daily activity levels can significantly impact TEE.

Measuring Physical Activity.   Ensuring that PA energy expenditure is accurately assessed is essential for providing appropriate energy recommendations for athletes. Looking at the female runner in the aforementioned scenario, failing to adjust her calorie intake to meet her daily needs could have adverse effects. This runner could end up overeating if she maintained a daily caloric intake comparable to what her needs are on a high activity day; alternatively, she could end up grossly undereating if she only consumed the amount of calories she needed for her low-activity days even on high-volume training days. This inflexible calorie consumption could have deleterious effects on her health and performance. Therefore, athletes must adjust their caloric intake according to daily fluctuations in PA, requiring the ability to estimate daily PA expenditure.

Indirect measures of energy expenditure. The best way to assess physical activity energy expenditure is to use indirect measures including indirect calorimetry via open-circuit spirometer and metabolic chamber. This process uses feedback from the individual including O_2 inhaled and CO_2 expired to measure energy expended during exercise. This can be done in a research or exercise physiology and biomechanics laboratory, or a portable metabolic cart can be used in the athlete's typical environment. In either scenario, when machines are calibrated and used appropriately, this can be a relatively accurate measurement of PA energy expenditure.

Metabolic equivalents of a tasks and the Compendium of Physical Activity. Physical activity questionnaires can be utilized as a way to assess daily physical activity levels. While there exist multiple physical activity questionnaires, many rely upon the Compendium of Physical Activities to provide an assessment of energy expenditure based upon the details of physical activity. Initially developed in 1989 and published in 1993, the Compendium of Physical Activities provides a coding scheme for various physical activities. These activities are then linked to the appropriate intensity level, which is measured by a metabolic equivalent of a task, or MET (Ainsworth et al. 2000). A MET is a ratio of the metabolic rate during a specific activity to a reference metabolic rate of 1.0 kilocalorie per kilogram per hour (1.0 kcal/kg/hr). METs are based on the measurement of oxygen consumption (mL per kilogram per minute, or, mL/kg/min), with the assumption that 1 MET equals the oxygen cost of sitting quietly of about 3.5 mL/kg/min.

The updated 2011 Compendium provides an extensive list of coded activities in different settings linked with their respective MET. This list is the most globally recognized set of values for METs and includes over 800 coded activities ranging from truck driving to ballroom dancing. The MET values range from 0.9 METs for sleeping to 23 METs for running 14.0 mph (Ainsworth et al. 2011). Based on the physical activity type and intensity per unit of time, METs can provide an estimate of energy expenditure. The equation factors in body weight, since an individual's weight affects caloric expenditure. The equation is as follows: MET × weight (kg) × duration (hours). So, remembering the 120 lb female runner identified earlier, let's say she ran 6.5 mph for 1.5 hours. The Compendium value for running at that speed in 12.8 METs. Using the equation, her energy expenditure while running would be: 12.8 METs × 54.5 kg × 1.5 hours = 1,047 kcal.

It is important to realize that MET values included in the Compendium, and most forms of physical activity energy expenditure measurements, include REE. That is, the 1,047 calories expended by the distance runner during her run is not just the energy needed for the activity of running, but includes the energy needed for the ongoing basal metabolic functions during this period of time. Thus, when calculating TEE by using estimates of energy expenditure for physical activity (such as METs), REE does not need to be added.

Using METs and the Compendium of Physical Activity has limitations as with any assessments using preestablished values to determine a measurement. One weakness with using METs is that the measurement assumes that all individuals expend 3.5 mL O_2/kg/min at rest, and this establishes the basis for other MET values. In actuality, this value may vary among individuals, such as someone who may only need 3.1 mL O_2/kg/min at rest, or conversely, someone may require 3.9 O_2/kg/min. This assumption that all individuals consume 3.5 mL O_2/kg/min could result in over- or underestimating energy expenditure, respectively. So, while MET values may not provide a precise value for energy expenditure, it can at least provide *relative* information. Looking at the example of the female distance runner, using METs it is estimated that she expends 1,047 calories during her 90-minute run. This value may not have high accuracy, but calculating METs for different durations and intensity (pace) she can get a gauge of her relative energy expenditure. Even considering its limitations, METs can provide a practical assessment tool for energy expenditure for various physical activities.

Measuring Total Daily Energy Expenditure

Many athletes need—or in some cases want—to know their TEE. This information is pertinent to weight management goals since it allows them to know what their food intake should be in order to lose, gain, or maintain their weight. Calculating TEE along with analyzing dietary intake also helps to assess where the athlete stands in regard to energy balance. Is the athlete's intake greater than, the same as, or less than their TEE? This information provides feedback to the athlete as to whether or not they are meeting the energy demands of their sport while maintaining overall health and immune function. Some of the most commonly employed techniques for measuring TEE are outlined as follows.

Doubly Labeled Water. Indirect calorimetry can be used to measure TEE, though this would require the individual to be confined to a metabolic chamber for a full day. This may not be realistic, nor would this represent daily energy expended in "real life." Due to the constraints of the equipment needed for metabolic cart measurement of energy expenditure, doubly labeled water was developed to assess energy expenditure in free-living individuals. In this method, an individual consumes water containing a measured, loaded dose of the stable isotopes of hydrogen, or deuterium ($^2H_2$), and oxygen, or ^{18}oxygen (^{18}O). The deuterium is eliminated as water, while the ^{18}O is eliminated as both H_2O and CO_2. The elimination rates of deuterium and ^{18}O are measured over time (by sampling saliva, urine, or blood), and the difference in these elimination rates measures the amount of CO_2 produced (not O_2 consumption as with metabolic carts). Carbon dioxide production can then be used to assess heat production, which provides a measurement of expended energy.

One advantage of doubly labeled water is that individuals are not limited by equipment allowing the measurement of athletes' energy expenditure in their own environments. The technique places minimal burden on the athlete other than needing to provide urine, saliva, or blood samples. Additionally, energy expenditure can be assessed over a period of up to 3 weeks. A major limitation of this method is that it is very expensive; moreover, it requires administration by a trained professional. Doubly labeled water measures TEE, but it cannot isolate and measure the energy expenditure of specific physical activities. Finally, doubly labeled water has an increased risk of error since it only measures CO_2 and does not measure O_2 consumption (Pinheiro Volp et al. 2011). Overall, though, when available, this method can be an ideal assessment in free-living individuals, and has been applied in research settings to validate other TEE measures.

Predictive Equations with an Activity Coefficient.   The equations outlined in Table 2.1 that measure REE can be multiplied by an activity coefficient, or activity factor, to estimate TEE. The activity coefficient is based on physical activity level, and so the practitioner needs to know the overall activity level of the individual. Table 2.2 shows activity coefficients commonly used.

The simplest way to calculate TEE is to determine an average activity coefficient for the day based on total activity. This coefficient is then multiplied by the REE calculated from the predictive equation. For example, a 165 lb male athlete was found to have an REE (using the Cunningham equation) of 1,620 kcal/day. This value would be multiplied by an activity coefficient of 2.1 for a heavy day of exercise. This is what this looks like:

1,620 kcal/day (REE) × 2.1 (activity coefficient) = 3,402 kcal/day

This method is only an estimate. Sports nutritionists and athletes must understand the limitations that come with using equations and that this value may under- or overestimate energy needs. Additionally, energy needs vary on a day-to-day basis and so, in most situations, an *average* TEE is calculated. This value may require daily adjustments according to variations in physical activity levels. This method provides a starting point for estimating TEE and can be fine-tuned according to feedback from anthropometric measures, as well as collecting feedback from the athlete regarding their energy levels and overall feeling.

Table 2.2 Activity coefficients

Approximate values for physical activity coefficients		
Activity level	**Average**	**Range**
Bed rest	1.2	1.1–1.3
Very sedentary	1.3	1.2–1.4
Light	1.5	1.4–1.6
Moderate	1.8	1.7–1.9
Heavy	2.1	1.9–2.3
Very heavy	2.3	2.0–2.6

Note: Approximate activity coefficients that when multiplied by REE can estimate TEE. While the middle column shows an average, it may be appropriate to use a value in the lower end of the range for females for better estimation.

Other measures of TEE include estimates that multiply a calorie value that is based on an activity by the weight (kg) of the individual. For example, a 55 kg female athlete who trains 5 days a week for several hours would need about 37 kcal/kg. Thus, her TEE, or energy needs, would be 55 kg × 37 kcal/kg/day = ~2,035 kcal/day. Table 2.3 shows an example of

Table 2.3 Estimated energy needs

Level of activity	Example of activity level	Energy expenditure, males (kcal/kg/day)	Energy expenditure, females (kcal/kg/day)
Sedentary (ADLs only)	Acute recovery from an injury	31	30
Moderate-intensity exercise 3–5 days per week or low-intensity short-duration training daily	Playing recreational soccer 1–1.5 hours every other day; practicing baseball or softball 2.5 hours daily 5 days a week	38	35
Training several hours a day 5 days a week	Swimming 1,000–10,000 m/day with resistance training; soccer practice including skills and conditioning training 2–3 hours a day	41	37
Rigorous training on an almost daily basis	Resistance training 10–15 hours per week such as a bodybuilder in a maintenance phase; swimming 7,000–17,000 m a day + 3 days of resistance training per week; typical training for college and elite-level football and basketball players	45	38–40
Extremely rigorous training	Training for a half or full ironman; running 15 miles a day or equivalent	51.5 and up to 60 or more	41 and up to 50 or more

Note: kcal/kg/day = kilocalorie per kilogram of body weight per day.
Source: Adapted from Macedonio and Dunford (2009).

estimated energy needs. These are the least accurate way to assess energy needs, though for individuals with limited access to other technology and computerized formulas, these provide a ballpark estimation that can be fine-tuned as needed.

An activity log can be used to better estimate energy expended as a result of planned training and exercise. Information should be gathered that includes daily, weekly, and even monthly variations in training intensity and duration for a thorough understanding of the athlete's energy needs; these concepts will be discussed in more detail in Chapter 5.

Other Forms of Technology.   There are many technological advances that allow total and physical activity energy expenditure measurements. Heart rate monitors have been used for some time with athletes to measure intensity levels of training, but they can also be used to estimate energy expenditure. Heart rate can estimate VO_2 and energy expenditure since it shows a linear relationship with these two variables at submaximal exercise. However, these devices are moderately reliable and can have a high margin of error, especially when it comes to measuring energy expenditure (Erdogan et al. 2010; Montgomery et al. 2009). Thus, these devices should be used for rough estimates only.

More recent technology has improved energy expenditure estimates. Accelerometers, a type of physical activity monitor, can sense physiological or mechanical responses to an individual's movement and these signals can be used to estimate physical activity energy expenditure. Information including the intensity, duration, and frequency of activity can be obtained; heart rate and heat produced by the body may also be measured and can be integrated in to the computation to provide more accurate energy estimation. These devices were initially used only in research settings due to the cost associated with the technology and advanced software; however, recent developments have resulted in accelerometers becoming available for commercial use that are much more affordable.

Accelerometers can be a convenient and noninvasive way to measure TEE in addition to estimating energy expended during physical activity. Some devices also provide other feedback such as assessing sleep quantity and quality, tracking steps taken, and measuring elevation. Yet, accelerometers should not be considered comparable to laboratory-based measures of energy expenditure, including indirect calorimetry and doubly labeled water. In a recent study looking at the reliability and validity of many of the most current devices found that they were only moderately accurate at estimating TEE with an error range of 12 to 29 percent (Ferguson et al. 2015). The devices were most likely to underestimate energy expenditure; thus, using these measurements to provide energy recommendations could result in an inadequate energy intake.

Finally, technological advancements that assist in the measurement of PA and TEE include various websites and "apps" (a software program or application). With the ubiquitous nature of the Internet, the majority of Americans have access to various websites that allow for estimation of energy expended through activity. Through the Internet individuals can access the predictive equations mentioned previously, such as the Harris–Benedict equation or Mifflin–St. Jeor equation to get an estimate of their TEE; the Internet would also allow individuals to access the METS Compendium to assess PA expenditure. There are also websites where individuals can enter in their age, height, weight, gender, and typical daily intake to get an estimate of their TEE. From there individuals enter information on specific PA performed and they can see not only an estimate of the energy expenditure for that activity, but they can also see how that affects their TEE. Common websites include www.myfitnesspal.com, www.loseit.com, and www.supertracker.usda.gov

Apps, as they have become commonly known, are software programs that are available on smartphones and other portable devices, and can also reference software that can be accessed when online. With so many Americans owning smartphones, apps on these devices can be a very accessible way to estimate activity energy expenditure. Most smartphones have accelerometers contained in them which allows for tracking of steps, and by mapping this information through a calibration algorithm a caloric value of energy expenditure is available to the user. Smartphones and other portable devices may also have sensors that detect body temperature changes and heart rate monitors as well as GPS capability to give more geographical details of the movement of an individual (such as altitude changes). Apps that integrate this information can provide more specific feedback to the individual including estimates of PA and TEE. The advantages of these technologies is that it provides regular and immediate information to the user. While technology is constantly advancing and accuracy continues to improve, the information provided from these technologies should still be considered estimates and not used as exact values.

There are many ways to measure TEE, and sports nutrition practitioners need to use the tools that are available to provide the best estimate. Doubly labeled water is considered the gold standard; though, for reasons previously described this assessment is not always practical. Other assessments of TEE include the use of Physical Activity Questionnaires and corresponding METs to add up expenditure throughout the day, predictive equations multiplied by an activity coefficient, and estimated energy needs using kcal/kg. For improved accuracy with any of these methods, details regarding the frequency, intensity, and duration of activity should be collected during the nutrition assessment. No method is without limitations, and it is up to the practitioner to determine which method is most appropriate based on available resources.

Definitions

Energy—the capacity to do work.

Joule—the SI unit of energy or work; equals the energy that is transferred when applying a force of one newton through a distance of one meter.

Resting energy expenditure (REE)—equivalent to resting metabolic rate (RMR); the amount of energy needed by the body at rest. Testing conditions are less stringent than BEE, which can result in a slightly higher value than BEE.

Basal energy expenditure (BEE)—equivalent to basal metabolic rate (BMR); the amount of energy needed by the body at complete rest. To be accurate, this must be measured in a postabsorptive state (the individual must not be actively digesting food and should be fasted more than 8 hours) and should be assessed immediately upon waking and before rising in the morning.

Adaptive thermogenesis—the decrease in energy expenditure beyond what could be predicted from body weight or its components as a result of a decrease in energy intake.

References

Ainsworth, B.E., W.L. Haskell, S.D. Herrmann, N. Meckes, D.R. Bassett Jr., C. Tudor-Locke, J.L. Greer, J. Vezina, M.C. Whitt-Glover, and A.S. Leon. 2011. "2011 Compendium of Physical Activities: A Second Update of Codes and MET Values." *Medicine and Science in Sports and Exercise* 43, no. 8, pp. 1575–81. doi:10.1249/MSS.0b013e31821ece12

Ainsworth, B.E., W.L. Haskell, M.C. Whitt, M.L. Irwin, A.M. Swartz, S.J. Strath, W.L. O'Brien, D.R. Bassett, Jr., K.H. Schmitz, P.O. Emplaincourt, D.R. Jacobs Jr., and A.S. Leon. 2000. "Compendium of Physical Activities: An Update of Activity Codes and MET Intensities." *Medicine and Science in Sports and Exercise* 32, no. 9 Suppl, pp. S498–504.

Cunningham, J.J. 1980. "A Reanalysis of the Factors Influencing Basal Metabolic Rate in Normal Adults." *American Journal of Clinical Nutrition* 33, no. 11, pp. 2372–74.

Erdogan, A., C. Cetin, H. Karatosun, and M.L. Baydar. 2010. "Accuracy of the Polar S810i(TM) Heart Rate Monitor and the Sensewear Pro Armband(TM) to Estimate Energy Expenditure of Indoor Rowing Exercise in Overweight and Obese Individuals." *Journal of Sports Science and Medicine* 9, no. 3, pp. 508–16.

Ferguson, T., A.V. Rowlands, T. Olds, and C. Maher. 2015. "The Validity of Consumer-Level, Activity Monitors in Healthy Adults Worn in Free-Living Conditions: A Cross-Sectional Study." *International Journal of Behavioral Nutrition and Physical Activity* 12, no. 1, p. 42. doi:10.1186/s12966-015-0201-9

Hall, K.D., S.B. Heymsfield, J.W. Kemnitz, S. Klein, D.A. Schoeller, and J.R. Speakman. 2012. "Energy Balance and Its Components: Implications for Body Weight Regulation." *The American Journal of Clinical Nutrition* 95, no. 4, pp. 989–94. doi:10.3945/ajcn.112.036350

Hasson, R.E., C.A. Howe, B.L. Jones, and P.S. Freedson. 2011. "Accuracy of Four Resting Metabolic Rate Prediction Equations: Effects of Sex, Body Mass Index, Age, and Race/Ethnicity." *Journal of Science and Medicine in Sport* 14, no. 4, pp. 344–51. doi:10.1016/j.jsams.2011.02.010

Macedonio, M.A., and M. Dunford. 2009. *The Athlete's Guide to Making Weight: Optimal Weight for Optimal Performance.* Champaign, IL: Human Kinetics.

Montgomery, P.G., D.J. Green, N. Etxebarria, D.B. Pyne, P.U. Saunders, and C.L. Minahan. 2009. "Validation of Heart Rate Monitor-Based Predictions of Oxygen Uptake and Energy Expenditure." *Journal of Strength and Conditioning Research* 23, no. 5, pp. 1489–95. doi:10.1519/JSC.0b013e3181a39277

Onur, S., V. Haas, A. Bosy-Westphal, M. Hauer, T. Paul, D. Nutzinger, H. Klein, and M.J. Muller. 2005. "L-Tri-Iodothyronine Is a Major Determinant of Resting Energy Expenditure in Underweight Patients with Anorexia Nervosa and During Weight Gain." *European Journal of Endocrinology* 152, no. 2, pp. 179–84. doi:10.1530/eje.1.01850

Oshima, S., S. Miyauchi, H. Kawano, T. Ishijima, M. Asaka, M. Taguchi, S. Torii, and M. Higuchi. 2011. "Fat-Free Mass Can Be Utilized to Assess Resting Energy Expenditure for Male Athletes of Different Body size." *Journal of Nutritional Science and Vitaminology (Tokyo)* 57, no. 6, pp. 394–400.

Pinheiro Volp, A.C., F.C. Esteves de Oliveira, R. Duarte Moreira Alves, E.A. Esteves, and J. Bressan. 2011. "Energy Expenditure: Components and Evaluation Methods." *Nutricion Hospitalaria* 26, no. 3, pp. 430–40. doi:10.1590/S0212-16112011000300002

Russell, J., L.A. Baur, P.J. Beumont, S. Byrnes, G. Gross, S. Touyz, S. Abraham, and S. Zipfel. 2001. "Altered Energy Metabolism in Anorexia Nervosa." *Psychoneuroendocrinology* 26, no. 1, pp. 51–63.

Taguchi, M., K. Ishikawa-Takata, W. Tatsuta, C. Katsuragi, C. Usui, S. Sakamoto, and M. Higuchi. 2011. "Resting Energy Expenditure Can Be Assessed by Fat-Free Mass in Female Athletes Regardless of Body Size." *Journal of Nutritional Science and Vitaminology (Tokyo)* 57, no. 1, pp. 22–29.

Tanner, R.E., L.B. Brunker, J. Agergaard, K.M. Barrows, R.A. Briggs, O.S. Kwon, L.M. Young, P.N. Hopkins, E. Volpi, R.L. Marcus, P.C. LaStayo, and M.J. Drummond. 2015. "Age-Related Differences in Lean Mass, Protein Synthesis and Skeletal Muscle Markers of Proteolysis After Bed Rest and Exercise Rehabilitation." *Journal of Physiology* 593, no. 18, pp. 4259–73. doi:10.1113/JP270699

Vogler, A.J., A.J. Rice, and C.J. Gore. 2010. "Validity and Reliability of the Cortex MetaMax3B Portable Metabolic System." *Journal of Sports Sciences* 28, no. 7, pp. 733–42. doi:10.1080/02640410903582776

Westerterp, K.R. 2004. "Diet Induced Thermogenesis." *Nutrition and Metabolism (Lond)* 1, no. 1, p. 5. doi:10.1186/1743-7075-1-5

CHAPTER 3

Energy Metabolism

Our bodies require adenine triphosphate (ATP) for muscular contraction, but we do not eat ATP, rather, we consume food. Thus, our bodies need to take the food that we eat and convert it into ATP, which is required for movement. The processes that make up this conversion are collectively referred to as energy metabolism. The three main macronutrients—carbohydrates, protein, and fat—are found in varying quantities in the foods we eat. Macronutrients contain energy, or calories, that can only be used or stored after digestion and absorption. If energy, in the form of ATP, is needed immediately, the body can use the metabolites from the breakdown of macronutrients to meet these needs. The three different energy systems that include the phosphagen system, glycolysis, and mitochondrial respiration provide ATP as an energy source for movement and muscular contraction. Thus, ATP is considered the energy currency of the cell.

The phosphagen system is anaerobic, meaning it does not need oxygen and provides rapid energy for maximal intensity exercise lasting 10 to 15 seconds. This system rapidly rephosphorylates ADP and Pi into ATP but can only be used for a very short period of time. Glycolysis is also an anaerobic energy system that can provide ATP quickly, for a slightly longer period than the phosphagen system, about 30 seconds. Mitochondrial respiration is an aerobic energy system, meaning it requires the presence of oxygen, and is the energy system used at rest and during exercise of low-to-moderate intensity.

While these are three distinct energy systems, they are interrelated in their contribution to exercise. Exercise duration, intensity, and an athlete's nutritional status will determine the contribution of each of these systems. Understanding the complex dynamic relationship between the three energy systems is essential for providing effective nutritional strategies for athletes to achieve optimal performance.

ATP: The Currency of the Cell

Recall the primary tenet of thermodynamics—energy cannot be created or destroyed. We consume energy from food in the form of macronutrients, which have chemical bonds that, when broken, release energy. Carbohydrates, fats, and, to a small degree, proteins, are broken down to provide energy that can be used immediately or stored as glycogen in the liver and muscle, and triglycerides in adipose tissues and intramuscular triglycerides. This stored energy is used to supply ATP, which takes energy in chemical form and transforms it into mechanical energy used for muscular contraction.

ATP is the basic unit of energy for all cells, and therefore is considered the currency of the cell (see Figure 3.1). ATP, a nucleoside triphosphate, contains a protein atom (adenine) and a sugar molecule (ribose), which are attached to three phosphate groups. The bonds connecting the last two phosphate groups are high-energy bonds. When these bonds are hydrolyzed through the action of the enzyme ATPase, energy is released and transferred to muscle cells energizing muscular activity.

Here you see the breakdown of ATP to ADP + Pi, with the cleavage of the bond between the ADP molecule and the last Pi releasing energy that powers muscular contraction. In order for work to continue, however, ADP needs to be rephosphorylated to ATP; that is, a phosphate group needs to be added to ADP to replenish ATP stores. The body only stores a limited amount of ATP (80 to 100 g, or, 3 oz), and only a percentage of ATP will be depleted during exercise in order to maintain basic cellular functioning (Baker, McCormick, and Robergs 2010). In fact, while total ATP stores remain relatively stable during exercise, there can

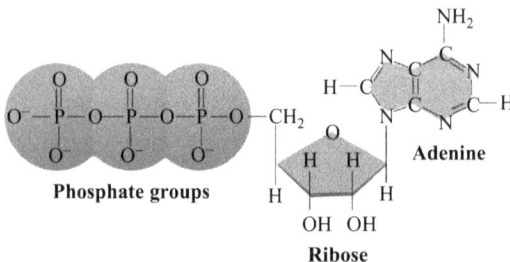

Figure 3.1 ATP: three phosphate groups, ribose, adenine

be a 1,000-fold increase in ATP demand. Consequently, there needs to be rapid turnover of ATP to continue supplying energy for movement of working muscle cells. Exercise lasting more than approximately five seconds requires ATP to be resynthesized. The body accomplishes this replenishment via three energy systems: two systems that produce small amounts of ATP quickly, lasting for a short duration, and a third system that replenishes large amounts of ATP over a long period of time.

Energy Systems

The Phosphagen System

The **phosphagen system**, also known as the phosphocreatine system, can replenish ATP quickly for a short duration (<10 seconds). A working muscle that has an extremely high energy demand will utilize phospho-creatine, or PCr. Creatine is a naturally occurring compound synthesized from arginine, glycine, and methionine, and the majority of the body's creatine pool is contained in the skeletal muscle in a phosphorylated form, phosphocreatine. Because PCr is a phosphorylated creatine mole-cule, it contains a high-energy phosphate bond. When a phosphate bond is hydrolyzed, a phosphate group is transferred to ADP to be replenished to ATP (see Figure 3.2).

Note that the arrow in this equation goes in both directions; that is, during periods of low activity or rest, ATP can be used to resynthesize creatine into creatine phosphate by donating a phosphate group.

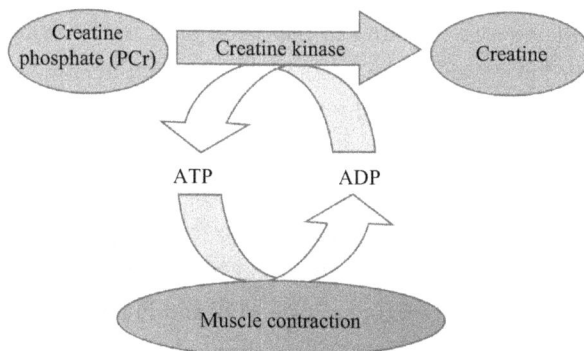

Figure 3.2 ADP + PCr (creatine kinase) ATP + Creatine

The breakdown of PCr does not require oxygen and since this system can replenish ATP rapidly, this system predominates at the onset of exercise, before oxygen uptake can meet energy demand, and during very-high-intensity exercise when the energy demand is extremely high. PCr is only available in limited quantities in skeletal muscle, so exercise relying upon the phosphagen system to replenish ATP only lasts 10 to 15 seconds at very high intensities (Baker, McCormick, and Robergs 2010). Examples include high-intensity, short-duration track and field events, resistance training, or a powerful golf swing. The phosphagen system may also predominate in the first several seconds of exercise lasting longer than 10 to 15 seconds, but another energy system is needed when ATP from the phosphagen system becomes depleted. Glycolysis is able to continue providing ATP when the phosphagen is exhausted.

Creatine can be consumed in the diet from protein-containing foods such as meat and fish; it can also be synthesized endogenously in the liver and pancreas. Most individuals rely upon dietary sources as well as endogenous synthesis to meet their creatine needs. Vegetarian diets are lower in creatine and thus vegetarian athletes tend to have lower creatine stores. Creatine supplementation will be discussed in Chapter 7.

Glycolysis

Because ATP produced from the phosphagen system is exhausted rapidly, continued replenishment of ATP relies upon **glycolysis**. Glycolysis is the breakdown of carbohydrate. All carbohydrate is digested and absorbed in the form of glucose or fructose. In the liver, fructose is converted into glucose. Glucose can be found in the blood or it can be stored in long chains, called glycogen, in the liver and the muscle. Either glycogen from the muscle or glucose from the blood can undergo glycolysis to yield ATP. Glycolysis takes place in the cytoplasm of the cell, and as with the phosphagen system, does not require oxygen. Glycolysis is initiated at the beginning of high-intensity exercise as is the phosphagen system, but because this process is more complex and requires additional enzymatically catalyzed steps to rephosphorylate ADP and Pi into ATP, it is not as rapid as the phosphagen system. While glycolysis does not replenish ATP as quickly as the phosphagen system, it can produce more total ATP. This is in part because skeletal muscle can store more glycogen than PCr.

Glycolysis is a process involving 10 enzymatically catalyzed reactions that ultimately results in the production of pyruvate. This process always begins with either glycogen stored directly in the muscle cell, or blood glucose that has been transported across the cell membrane and into the cytoplasm. The end product of glycolysis, pyruvate, has two potential fates and it is the energy demand of the cell that determines whether pyruvate will be (1) transported into the mitochondria and converted into acetyl-CoA or (2) converted into lactic acid. If the energy demands of the cell cannot be met through oxidative metabolism, or if the muscle fiber is highly glycolytic (type 2 fiber), then pyruvate will be converted to lactic acid, which quickly disassociates into lactate and a H+ ion. High-intensity exercise such as a 200 m sprint or a set of 10 power cleans are examples of activities that would heavily rely on ATP produced by glycolysis. This process is sometimes referred to as "fast glycolysis," or "anaerobic glycolysis," which is somewhat of a misnomer since all glycolysis is anaerobic. "Fast glycolysis" is somewhat more telling, in that when rate of glycolysis is high, most pyruvate formed will be converted to lactic acid because insufficient oxygen is available within the mitochondria to keep pace with the entry of acetyl-CoA; basically there is a "traffic jam" of substrate so pyruvate must be diverted from the mitochondria (by being converted into lactic acid).

If the energy demand of the cell is lower and ATP requirements can be met through the complete oxidative metabolism of glucose, pyruvate is shuttled into mitochondria to be converted into acetyl-CoA, which then enters the Krebs Cycle, a process sometimes referred to as "aerobic glycolysis" or "slow glycolysis." These terms are also misnomers since many amino acids and all fatty acids are converted into acetyl-CoA before entry into the Krebs cycle and eventually the electron transport chain (ETC). In reality, glycolysis ends in the cytosol of the cell with the production of pyruvate, which is then converted into acetyl Co-A for further metabolism, or lactic acid, which then disassociates into lactate and a H+ ion. However, for the sake of simplicity, it is easiest to think of the metabolism of glucose as being either incomplete (pyruvate is converted into lactic acid, also known as "fast" glycolysis), or complete (pyruvate is shuttled to the mitochondria to be converted to acetyl Co-A, which then enters the Krebs cycle for complete metabolism, also known as "slow" glycolysis. Once pyruvate enters the Krebs cycle, it undergoes a completely different pathway and is no longer glycolysis. See Figure 3.3).

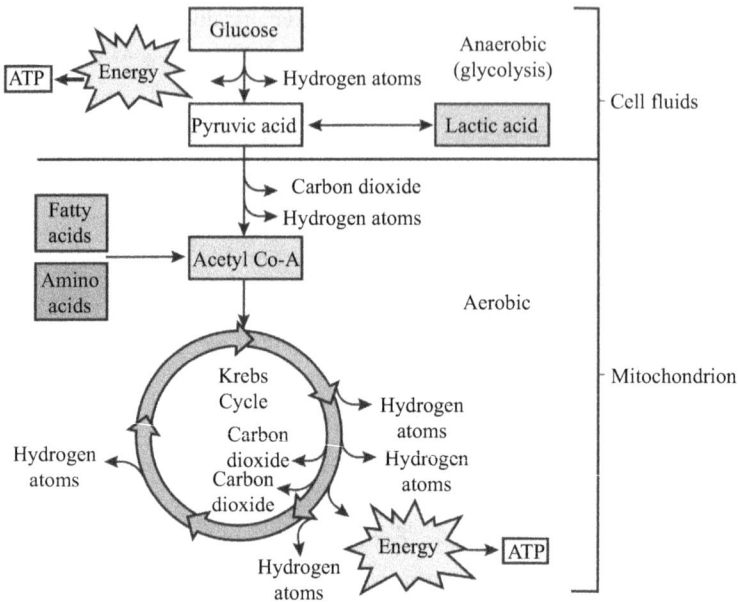

Figure 3.3 Summary of glycolysis and Krebs cycle

Glycolysis is the primary source of the ATP that is required for a maximal bout lasting around 30 seconds, with the phosphagen system contributing smaller amounts of ATP over this period (Baker, McCormick, and Robergs 2010). Sport examples relying primarily upon glycolysis include a 50 m sprint in swimming, a 200 to 400 m running sprint, or soccer and basketball players engaging in repeated, high-intensity intervals up and down the soccer field or basketball court.

While the production of ATP is rapid via "incomplete" or "fast" glycolysis, and storage of glycogen has not yet been depleted, this energy system cannot be used as the primary source of ATP for sustained activity. First, incomplete or fast glycolysis that converts pyruvate to lactate can produce ATP more rapidly but will only yield two ATPs. However, when pyruvate is converted to lactic acid, it quickly dissociates into lactate and an H+ ion. Lactate can be used by the liver as a fuel source or converted into glucose (Cori cycle); but the H+ ion that is produced from ATP hydrolysis reactions decreases the pH of the cell and slows enzymatic reactions. Athletes often "feel" this acidification of the body and refer to it as the "burn" or "build-up of lactic acid." Thus, it is not lactic acid itself that causes fatigue but rather the acidosis that results from the hydrogen ions that are produced from a number of reactions, most notably the hydrolysis of ATP. When pH drops, respiratory rate increases exponentially in an effort to buffer the hydrogen being produced. However, exhaled CO_2 is not nearly as acidic as hydrogen and eventually exercise intensity must decrease precipitously because hydrogen directly impairs the muscle's ability to contract.

Mitochondrial Respiration (Oxidative Metabolism)

Mitochondrial respiration, also known as oxidative metabolism or aerobic metabolism, meets ATP demand at rest and during low-intensity exercise. Even during extremely high-intensity exercise, some cells (such as cardiac cells) can *only* use energy produced from aerobic metabolism. Aerobic metabolism completes the transfer of energy from the breakdown of carbohydrate, fats, and proteins from the foods we eat into the energy we need to maintain life. Before these macronutrients can be completely metabolized by the Krebs cycle and ETC, they must undergo preliminary metabolic steps. The following will give a brief overview of how each macronutrient is metabolized in a series of catabolic reactions that eventually produce energy and heat, as well as the metabolic by-products: water and carbon dioxide.

The pyruvate produced from glycolysis is converted to acetyl-CoA, and it enters the Krebs cycle (or TCA cycle or Citric acid cycle), an irreversible step. For each glucose molecule that enters glycolysis, two pyruvate molecules are formed, each can enter into the Krebs cycle given there is adequate oxygen. Ultimately, from the Krebs cycle, each molecule of glucose produces two ATP and ten hydrogen ions. Because these hydrogen ions are unstable, they are immediately bound to a nicotinamide adenine dinucleotide (NAD) or flavin adenine dinucleotide (FAD) molecule, thus becoming NADH and $FADH_2$. The resulting six NADH and two $FADH_2$ molecules then "carry" the electrons to the ETC within the mitochondrial membrane matrix. Once the hydrogen ions are removed, the NAD and FAD carriers can "pick up" additional electrons generated by the Krebs cycle. Within the ETC, hydrogen ions are sent through a series of oxidation-reduction, or **redox reactions**, within linked specialized complexes called cytochromes. As hydrogen molecules are "pumped" through the cytochromes, potential energy is stored in what can simply be thought of as a hydrogen reservoir. When the stored hydrogen molecules move down through the final cytochrome, there is an electrochemical gradient from which energy is captured and used to rephosphorylate ADP and Pi into ATP via the enzyme ATP synthase. Oxygen then combines with the free hydrogen ions to produce water (thus the requirement for oxygen). If oxygen is unavailable, the aforementioned metabolic reactions could not continue because the free hydrogen ions would quickly drop the pH of the cell and cause cessation of enzymatic activity (cellular death). The result is the production of 32 ATP from the ETC, and a total production of 36 ATP from the complete metabolism of one molecule of glucose.

Fats can also be used as a substrate for the oxidative energy system and, to a lesser degree, so can protein. Triglycerides in fat cells can be broken down through enzymatic action that releases free fatty acids into the blood, which can eventually be taken up by muscle cells. There are also limited amounts of triglycerides stored in the muscle that can be broken down into free fatty acids. Through a process called beta oxidation, free fatty acids that have entered the mitochondria are broken down. The result is the production of acetyl-CoA that enters the Krebs cycle, and hydrogen ions that are carried by NADH and $FADH_2$ to the ETC. The energy yield from one triglyceride molecule is significantly greater than that of one molecule of glucose. The actual number of ATP produced depends upon the number of carbons in the triglyceride. As an example, a triglyceride containing three 18-carbon fatty acids will yield 463 molecules of ATP (22 ATP from the oxidation of glycerol, + 147 ATP per fatty acid × 3)! This is almost 13 times the amount of ATP produced from one glucose molecule. While the production takes much longer, the yield is significantly greater.

The oxidation of protein is a less-efficient process and therefore protein is not an ideal energy substrate. Some amino acids resulting from the breakdown of protein known as glucogenic amino acids can be converted into glucose via a process called gluconeogenesis, which then can be oxidized. There are ketogenic amino acids that can be broken down to acetyl-CoA and thus can be used in the Krebs cycle or can be used to produce ketones. While this process will be discussed in further detail in Chapter 4, it should be understood that protein is an inefficient source of energy and contributes minimally to short-term exercise, and about 5 to 10 percent of energy (and up to 18 percent) to prolonged exercise.

The three energy systems, the phosphagen system, glycolysis, and mitochondrial respiration, are significantly more complex than what is explained in the aforementioned descriptions. To truly have a thorough understanding of energy metabolism, knowledge of exercise physiology or nutritional biochemistry or both is required. For the purpose of this text, this brief overview is sufficient to illustrate the overall concept that the energy demands of the body determine the energy system(s) that are called upon, as well as the need to consume the appropriate nutrients to supply substrates for these systems and how these three systems are interrelated.

The Three Energy Systems Work in Concert to Provide Energy for Activity

While the three energy systems appear to be distinct, it is important to understand they are interrelated and work together to contribute to energy required for exercise. Regardless of the type or intensity of the activity, all three energy systems produce ATP to meet energy demands. It is also important to consider that energy demands may differ throughout the body. For example, when performing maximal cycling sprints, ATP demand in the muscle cells of the quadriceps will be very high and primarily met through the phosphagen system and fast or incomplete glycolysis; however, energy demands of the biceps are probably much lower, therefore aerobic metabolism will be the primary ATP contributor.

Duration of the exercise activity is an important consideration for which energy system predominates. The phosphagen system is the immediate source of energy for high-intensity exercise, yet, is depleted quickly. Glycolysis does not provide ATP as rapidly at the phosphagen system, but it too is initiated at the onset of exercise, and after 10 seconds will be the primary contributor of energy for up to two minutes. Mitochondrial respiration is always being used at rest and rate of ATP production via this pathway increases at the onset of exercise, regardless of other contributors of ATP; however, it becomes the main energy source when exercise lasts longer than 75 seconds and continues to supply ATP indefinitely (albeit rate of ATP production can decrease and exercise capacity can diminish) (Baker, McCormick, and Robergs 2010). Even during long-duration exercise, the phosphagen system and fast glycolysis will continue to contribute small amounts of ATP. Ultimately, the production of ATP from all three systems allows the energy from food to fuel muscle contraction and exercise.

Fuel Substrate Utilization

Fuel Substrate Utilization

The three energy systems illustrate the mechanisms by which energy is provided at different intensities and duration of exercise. Yet the picture is incomplete without seeing how fuel substrate not only supplies energy for activity, but also becomes the limiting factor for exercise duration and intensity. Understanding the importance of how food contributes to sustaining power output and delaying fatigue is essential for making appropriate dietary recommendations for athletes.

Think of a dimmer switch as an analogy for fuel substrate utilization. At low-intensity exercise, when there is sufficient oxygen, mitochondrial respiration predominates. Fat (fatty acids) is the primary energy source for ATP production, though some amount of carbohydrate is required to regenerate intermediates of the Krebs cycle. As exercise intensity increases, the rate of demand for ATP increases beyond what can be supplied by fat. This is primarily due to limited oxygen availability and blood flow, as well as other negative feedback mechanisms produced from metabolic intermediates that inhibit the enzymes involved in mitochondrial respiration. Additionally, fat is a dense molecule and must undergo a time-consuming process known as beta-oxidation before it can be converted into acetyl-CoA and enter into Krebs cycle. Because glucose (or glycogen) undergoes far fewer steps before entry into the Krebs cycle, it can be metabolized aerobically to yield ATP much more quickly than fat. If exercise intensity is to increase further, rate of ATP rephosphorylation must also increase. *Absolute* fat oxidation will continue to increase up to a point; however, its *relative* contribution will decrease. Therefore, other metabolic pathways (fast glycolysis and PCr) will have to contribute to meet ATP demand. Thus, it is the energy demand of the working cells that are required to maintain or increase a given power output or rate of muscle contraction that determines which energy system is utilized.

Importantly, during high-intensity aerobic and anaerobic exercise, carbohydrate is the main source of fuel at higher intensities. This "fuel" will ultimately be used for ATP generation, which is directly involved in muscle contraction. The faster ATP can be generated the faster the muscle will contract. Fat will still supply some energy for exercise but the amount will be much less. Fat will also be used for much of the energy needed by inactive muscles and not the organs (heart, kidneys, stomach, etc.). So, while all three systems are active simultaneously, their relative contribution will vary according to exercise intensity and metabolic involvement in the exercise task.

Knowing that intensity determines which energy system and, consequently, which fuel source (fat, carbohydrate, or both) sustains activity, it is essential to be able to measure exercise intensity in order to provide appropriate nutrition recommendations. Heart rate can be used to measure exercise intensity, though the most precise measurement is volume of oxygen consumption (VO_2). VO_2 is the volume of oxygen consumed per minute per unit of body mass (mL/min/kg), and measures the metabolic demand of exercise. One's maximal VO_2, or **VO_2 max**, is a measure of one's cardiorespiratory fitness, or, generally speaking, is used as a measure of one's aerobic capacity. VO_2 max is the highest intensity of exercise that can be sustained aerobically. VO_2 max can be measured using indirect calorimetry methods such as an open circuit spirometer or "metabolic cart," as described in Chapter 2.

Aerobic exercise intensity can be expressed as a percentage relative to one's VO_2 max. For example, "low exercise intensity" relative to one's maximal aerobic capacity corresponds to approximately 30 percent or less of VO_2 max. At this intensity, individuals are utilizing mostly fat to meet energy demands. At moderate-intensity exercise, the relative contribution of fat and carbohydrate used to meet ATP demands are roughly equal (about 50 to 50). At vigorous or high exercise intensity such as 70 percent of VO_2 max or greater, carbohydrate is the greatest contributor of energy used to meet ATP demands. See Figure 3.4 illustrating this concept.

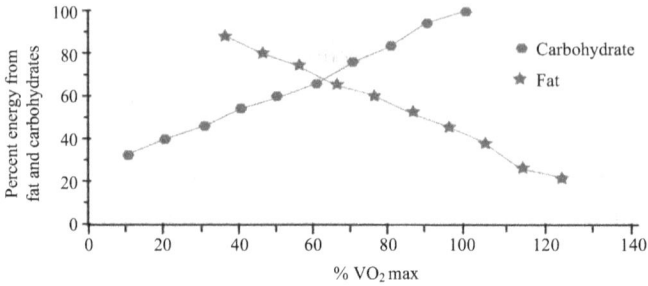

At low exercise intensity as defined by percentage of VO_2 max, fat predominates as an energy source. At moderate intensity exercise relative contributions of fat and carbohydrate are equal. At high intensity exercise carbohydrate contributes relatively more energy.

Figure 3.4 Contribution of carbohydrate and fat relative to exercise intensity

If adequate carbohydrate is unavailable, fat must be used, albeit at a much slower rate, to meet ATP demands. In a scenario such as this, athletes risk "hitting the wall" or "bonking." This is the experience of extreme reduction in aerobic power output and inability to maintain a given pace. It is often experienced by endurance athletes at some point in their career and is a result of insufficient carbohydrate availability. Even in the presence of adequate oxygen and fat stores, when carbohydrate, or glycogen, stores are depleted, exercise intensity suffers dramatically.

It is important to remember when discussing carbohydrate and fat contribution at different percentages of exercise intensity, *relative* contribution is what is being referenced. For example, relative contribution of fat and carbohydrate at 65 percent of one's VO_2 max is approximately equal, about 50 percent. However, this is distinct from absolute contribution. At low intensity, fat predominates as an energy source, yet the absolute rate of oxidation is only moderate, approximately 26 μmol/kg/min (a unit of measurement for fat oxidation) (Melzer 2011). At 65 percent of one's VO_2 max, when relative contribution of fat is only 50 percent, the absolute rate of fat oxidation is maximal, ~40 μmol/kg/min. So, even though the percentage of contribution of fat as an energy source is higher at lower intensities, the absolute fat oxidation is actually less than that at moderate exercise intensities.

The Myth of the "Fat Burning Zone"

Understanding the difference between *relative* and *absolute* rates of oxidation demonstrates why the "fat burning zone" is misleading in terms of weight loss. Many cardiovascular exercise machines, such as treadmills, elliptical machines, and recumbent bicycles show a "fat burning" zone promoting greater fat burning capacity at lower intensities. While fat provides *relatively* greater energy contribution at lower intensities, *absolute* fat burning is greatest at moderate intensities. Further, at high intensities, fat contributes relatively less energy, but total caloric expenditure is greatest (which is probably more important when trying to lose weight). While this will be discussed further in Chapter 8, which examines weight management, for now keep in mind that exercising in the fat burning zone may not prove to be an effective weight loss strategy.

Intensity is not the only variable that modulates fuel substrate utilization during exercise. Training status, exercise duration, and composition of the diet also affect the relative and absolute contribution of carbohydrate and fat to energy metabolism (Gonzalez and Stevenson 2012). Looking at training status, it has been shown that endurance training increases whole body rates of fat oxidation and decreases the rate of carbohydrate oxidation at both relative and absolute exercise intensities (Yeo et al. 2011). Specifically, endurance training increases mitochondrial volume allowing for greater fat oxidation and decreases activation of carbohydrate metabolism, with the result of sparing glycogen (Yeo et al. 2011). Glycogen sparing has significant performance benefits and is often a goal of endurance athletes. Any amount of glycogen that can be spared, or reserved, prevents insufficient glycogen availability from becoming the limiting factor in intensity or duration or both. Remember, the body has almost limitless fat stores but only limited stores of glycogen. The effect of these glycogen-sparing adaptations is that athletes rely upon great fat oxidation at given exercise intensities, potentially allowing athletes to train harder or longer with greater carbohydrate availability. Training status will also increase glycogen capacity, as well as the body's ability to utilize carbohydrate and lactate. This will be discussed in Chapter 6 in "Carbohydrate Loading."

Recent research has focused on dietary manipulations to increase fat oxidation with the hopes of sparing muscle glycogen. In fact, fat oxidation can be altered through specific nutritional strategies. Research has shown that increased fat intake (as a percentage of normal daily kcal or absolute increases beyond normal diet) increases fat oxidation and downregulates carbohydrate metabolism (Spriet 2014). Additionally, decreased carbohydrate availability increases the rate of fat oxidation at any given exercise intensity (Spriet 2014). Decreased CHO availability can be the result of depleted glycogen stores from exhaustive exercise, or due to insufficient dietary intake of CHO (purposefully or accidentally). Multiple adaptations occur on a cellular level that explain this shift in fuel substrate utilization. Adaptations that increase utilization of fat during exercise include improved fat transport into the mitochondria and enhanced regulation of intramuscular triglyceride synthesis and breakdown, and upregulation of enzymes involved in fat metabolism (Spriet 2014).

These cellular adaptations have prompted questions regarding optimal fuel sources for endurance exercise. There have been investigations to determine if athletes should be encouraged to have a higher fat–lower carbohydrate intake to promote greater fat oxidation, spare glycogen, and ultimately improve performance. Before these findings can be translated to revised nutrition and dietary strategies for performance, more research is needed. While research supports that dietary and training manipulations can increase fat oxidation at given exercise intensity, there is insufficient support that there are performance benefits to these strategies. Athletes may be able to increase fat utilization to a greater extent at higher exercise intensities, but the evidence is lacking that this results in performance benefits (Hawley et al. 2011; Ormsbee, Bach, and Baur 2014; Yeo et al. 2011). Rather, research has consistently shown an **ergogenic effect** when carbohydrate is consumed before and during exercise at given intensities and durations (Burke et al. 2011; Cermak and van Loon 2013; Lima-Silva et al. 2013). The benefits of carbohydrate intake before, during, and after exercise will be discussed further in Chapter 4 on Nutrient Recommendations.

Understanding the concept "fuel substrate utilization" at various exercise intensities illustrates the importance of providing proper nutrition strategies. The body has almost endless fat stores, even in very lean athletes. This reliance upon fat at low intensity is what allows endurance athletes such as long-distance runners and cyclists to exercise for hours. Yet, even these athletes rely upon carbohydrate because, in order to metabolize fat, carbohydrates are required. As intensity increases, so does reliance upon carbohydrate, yet the body has limited carbohydrate storage capacity. Endogenous stores of carbohydrate (blood glucose, muscle, and liver glycogen) can become depleted during long-duration exercise, and thus the body becomes reliant upon exogenous sources (= consumption of carbohydrate from food and beverages).

While inadequate nutrition becomes a limiting factor in exercise, appropriate nutrition practices will sustain activity and enhance performance. This will be discussed in further detail in "Nutrient Recommendations." The concept of the dimmer switch is essential for providing the best nutrient recommendations for athletes. Knowing which fuel substrates will be called upon, and which energy systems predominate when, will be necessary for ensuring dietary intake of optimal food sources.

Definitions

Phosphagen system—This provides an immediate and limited supply of ATP by donating high-energy phosphate compounds.

Glycolysis—It is the metabolic pathway using glucose to produce pyruvate and energy through the replenishment of ATP.

Mitochondrial respiration—It is a series of catabolic reactions transpiring in the mitochondria of the cell, requiring oxygen, with the result of producing large amounts of ATP to be used for energy production.

Redox reactions—It is a chemical reaction where the transfer of electrons between substances results in a change in the oxidation state of atoms.

VO$_2$ max—It is the maximum volume of oxygen that can be taken in during one minute of exhaustive exercise; often used as a measure of aerobic capacity.

Ergogenic—It is performance enhancing. An ergogenic aid is an external influence enhancing athletic performance, and may include performance enhancing drugs, dietary supplements, and physiological, mechanical, or psychological aids.

References

Baker, J.S., M.C. McCormick, and R.A. Robergs. 2010. "Interaction Among Skeletal Muscle Metabolic Energy Systems During Intense Exercise." *Journal of Nutrition and Metabolism* 2010, pp. 1–13. doi:10.1155/2010/905612

Burke, L.M., J.A. Hawley, S.H. Wong, and A.E. Jeukendrup. 2011. "Carbohydrates for Training and Competition." *Journal of Sports Sciences* 29, Suppl 1, pp. S17–27. doi:10.1080/02640414.2011.585473

Cermak, N.M., and L.J. van Loon. 2013. "The Use of Carbohydrates During Exercise as an Ergogenic Aid." *Sports Medicine* 43, no. 11, pp. 1139–55. doi:10.1007/s40279-013-0079-0

Gonzalez, J.T., and E.J. Stevenson. 2012. "New Perspectives on Nutritional Interventions to Augment Lipid Utilisation During Exercise." *British Journal of Nutrition* 107, no. 3, pp. 339–49. doi:10.1017/S0007114511006684

Hawley, J.A., L.M. Burke, S.M. Phillips, and L.L. Spriet. 2011. "Nutritional Modulation of Training-Induced Skeletal Muscle Adaptations." *Journal of Applied Physiology* 110, no. 3, pp. 834–45. doi:10.1152/japplphysiol.00949.2010

Lima-Silva, A.E., F.O. Pires, R. Bertuzzi, M.D. Silva-Cavalcante, R.S. Oliveira, M.A. Kiss, and D. Bishop. 2013. "Effects of a Low- or a High-Carbohydrate Diet on Performance, Energy System Contribution, and Metabolic Responses During Supramaximal Exercise." *Applied Physiology, Nutrition, and Metabolism* 38, no. 9, pp. 928–34. doi:10.1139/apnm-2012-0467

Melzer, K. 2011. "Carbohydrate and Fat Utilization During Rest and Physical Activity." *European Society for Clinical Nutrition and Metabolism* 6, p. 8.

Ormsbee, M.J., C.W. Bach, and D.A. Baur. 2014. "Pre-Exercise Nutrition: The Role of Macronutrients, Modified Starches and Supplements on Metabolism and Eendurance Performance." *Nutrients* 6, no. 5, pp. 1782–808. doi:10.3390/nu6051782

Spriet, L.L. 2014. "New Insights into the Interaction of Carbohydrate and Fat Metabolism During Exercise." *Sports Medicine* 44, no. Suppl 1, pp. S87–96. doi:10.1007/s40279-014-0154-1

Yeo, W.K., A.L. Carey, L. Burke, L.L. Spriet, and J.A. Hawley. 2011. "Fat Adaptation in Well-Trained Athletes: Effects on Cell Metabolism." *Applied Physiology, Nutrition, and Metabolism* 36, no. 1, pp. 12–22. doi:10.1139/H10-089

CHAPTER 4

The Building Blocks of Sports Nutrition: Carbohydrate, Protein, Fat, and Hydration

Food is fuel. The foods we consume are composed of three macronutrients responsible for supplying energy to the body for physical activity. All energy used by the body is derived from the food we eat. Carbohydrate, protein, and fat are the three macronutrients found in foods providing calories and thus supply the energy that fuels performance, yet their contribution to energy production is not equal. Knowing the basic structure and metabolism of these three macronutrients allows for a better understanding of their function in the body. General functions of these nutrients will be outlined, and more specifically, the role of carbohydrate, protein, and fat as it pertains to exercise and activity. This chapter identifies food sources of these nutrients that contribute to optimal health and performance. Fluids are a fourth nutrient essential for optimal health as well as for supporting athletic performance. In this chapter, hydration needs of the athlete will be discussed as well as methods to assess hydration status.

Sports nutritionists have a unique role in bridging the gap between science and implementation of evidence-based recommendations. Extensive research has developed a set of evidence-based practices to help athletes optimize their performance, though research continues to evolve and these recommendations are far from static. One of the primary tenets of sports nutrition relates to carbohydrate intake; as this is the primary source of energy for high-intensity training, athletes need to be educated on the importance of consuming enough carbohydrate, and at the appropriate time. Protein intake and timing of intake is also important, considering its role relative to skeletal muscle adaptation and recovery from exercise. Stored body fat and dietary triglycerides serve as an energy source at rest and during low-intensity exercise. Dietary fat is also required for the absorption of fat-soluble vitamins. However, athletes should be wary of consuming too much fat as it can displace dietary carbohydrate and protein. Athletes must also pay attention to hydration status and maintain euhydration. Hydration needs can be met in numerous ways, and best hydration practices are still being investigated. It is important to consider these recommendations within the context of a meal plan and not as isolated components, and the sports nutritionist needs to integrate these nutrients in a consequential and practical way.

Translating available research on nutrition for sport and activity and applying it in a meaningful way to athletes is an art as much as it is a science. Nutrition has profound effects on performance, from providing fuel for muscular contraction and movement, to supplying the brain with adequate fuel so that it can focus, concentrate, and strategize. Nutritional strategies can ensure that physical training yields growth of lean muscle mass and increased cardiovascular capacity. It is through nutritional practices that one achieves desired body composition changes. Nutrition has a considerable impact on overall health and immune functioning, which allows athletes to continue to train and avoid unnecessary periods of illness.

Overall, following effective nutrition recommendations supports athletes in realizing their athletic potential. Yet, these benefits are only seen if athletes have been educated on the best practices of sport nutrition. Athletes must then practice effective nutrition strategies on a daily basis through training and develop a fine-tuned game plan for implementation on race day.

Carbohydrates

Structure, Basic Functions, and Food Forms

Chemically, carbohydrates are molecules composed of carbon (C), hydrogen (H), and oxygen (O) atoms, thus giving carbohydrate its abbreviation of CHO. As previously described, carbohydrates provide approximately four kilocalories, or calories, per gram, a measure of its potential energy.

Carbohydrates are classified according to their chemical structure. Simple carbohydrates are composed of one sugar molecule (glucose, fructose, and galactose) known as monosaccharides (saccharide means sugar), or two sugar molecules (sucrose, maltose, and lactose) known as disaccharides. Fruits, vegetables, dairy products such as milk and yogurt, and table sugar are all dietary sources of simple carbohydrates. Many sports nutrition products, such as gels and sports drinks, are also composed largely of simple carbohydrates. Complex carbohydrates are composed of more than two sugar molecules found in linear or branched chain forms. These include starch, a glucose polymer found in plants, and glycogen, the storage form of glucose polymers in animals (including humans). Complex carbohydrates in the diet are found in legumes; starchy vegetables such as peas, corn, and potatoes; and grains. The digestion of complex carbohydrates takes longer than simple carbohydrates due to greater enzymatic action. Minimally processed complex carbohydrates are an important source of dietary fiber in addition to their provision of energy.

Carbohydrates are sometimes dichotomized as "good" or "bad," but this overly simplistic view of carbohydrates does not illustrate the diverse nature of this nutrient. It is erroneous to say that simple carbohydrates are bad for us and complex carbohydrates are good. For example, it would be difficult to argue that an apple, a simple carbohydrate, is unhealthy. A more precise approach looks at the nutrients that the carbohydrate food provides, the amount that is consumed, and, for an athlete, the timing of intake. Individuals, including athletes, are encouraged to focus on nutrient-rich forms of carbohydrates that include fruits, vegetables (starchy and nonstarchy), whole grains, milk, yogurt, and legumes. These foods will contribute essential vitamins, minerals, fiber, in addition to the energy they provide, and should comprise the foundation of an athlete's diet. Most of an athlete's energy will come from complex carbohydrates, though simple carbohydrates such as fruits and vegetables are also essential.

Processed foods made with refined grains and added sugars contribute energy but may offer little nutritional value regarding its nutrient profile, and thus their intake should be limited. These include snacks such as chips, crackers, cookies, and other commercial baked goods; sodas and sweetened drinks; and other white grains and sugar cereals. That being said, there are instances where simple, and slightly more processed carbohydrates may be appropriate for athletes and can be included in the diet, such as right before or during exercise. Timing of nutrient intake will be discussed later in this chapter.

Fiber

Fiber is an indigestible form of carbohydrate including polysaccharides, oligosaccharides, lignin, and other plant components. The human body lacks the enzymes to digest the components in fiber, but it is far from an inert substance. Dietary fibers are often classified as soluble and insoluble. Soluble fiber dissolves in water, thus attracting water and forming a gel, and slows digestion, creating a feeling of fullness. Food sources of soluble fiber include apples, blueberries, oats, nuts, and beans. Insoluble fiber can have a laxative effect and adds bulk to fecal matter, helping to prevent constipation. Whole wheat and other whole grains, cruciferous vegetables like broccoli and cauliflower, dark leafy greens, and grapes are all sources of insoluble fiber. Getting adequate fiber in the diet is associated with overall health benefits, though foods that have "added" fiber such as chicory root or psyllium are not known to have the same health benefits as foods with naturally occurring fiber. These foods may also cause gastrointestinal (GI) distress in some individuals. Thus, it is best to educate athletes on obtaining fiber from natural foods including fruits, vegetables, whole grains, and legumes.

Glycemic Index

Carbohydrates can also be classified according to the body's glycemic response to carbohydrate-containing foods. That is, glycemic index is the rise in blood glucose level over baseline over a 2-hour period following consumption of a specified amount of carbohydrate (usually 50 g). This is then compared to the blood glucose response to the same amount of a reference food (usually either glucose or white bread). A numerical value is assigned to this food and allows comparison of various carbohydrate foods and how they impact blood glucose levels. Because we typically do not consume foods in isolation, using the glycemic index is not usually practical and has obvious limitations. The concept of glycemic *load* has been established to factor in both quantity and quality of the carbohydrate in question. Glycemic load equals the grams of carbohydrate in a serving of a food times the glycemic index. For example, watermelon has a high glycemic index, though contains few grams of carbohydrate per serving. Thus, the effect of this high glycemic index food on blood glucose might not be as great as a food with a high glycemic index *and* has more grams of carbohydrate per serving. However, what is not accounted for here is the effect of other nutrients of other foods that are eaten at the same meal. Consuming protein-containing food along with a high glycemic index food will mitigate the effect on blood glucose.

Use of the glycemic index and glycemic load as a way to characterize the quality of carbohydrates is controversial. There lacks standardization of how glycemic index values are tested and measured, as well as variability of the glycemic index in the foods themselves (including relation to where they were grown, how they were processed, and cooking methods). There is variability between individuals' blood glucose response to a given food; this is just to name a few of the concerns with using glycemic index or load as a measure of carbohydrate quality. Regardless, research has demonstrated the damaging role elevated blood glucose levels have on the development of chronic diseases, including obesity and diabetes. There are considerable health implications for understanding glycemic index and glycemic load that are outside of the scope of this text. As it pertains to exercise, glycemic index has limited application for athletes and the timing of nutrient intake as we will see in the following section on carbohydrate recommendations.

Carbohydrate Metabolism

When individuals consume carbohydrate-containing foods, the carbohydrate portion is digested via enzymatic action and is ultimately released as glucose in the blood. The pancreas senses increased levels of glucose in the blood and releases insulin to promote the cellular uptake of glucose to meet immediate energy needs while maintaining homeostatic balance of glucose in the blood (between 70 and 110 mg/dL). The remaining glucose gets stored. Through **glycogenesis**, glucose gets stored with water as glycogen as a stored form of energy, though the amount that can be stored is limited. Most glycogen is stored in the muscle (about 300 to 400 g), while some amount is also stored in the liver to help regulate blood glucose (70 to 100 g). These amounts can be altered slightly through training and dietary manipulation, as will be discussed in Chapter 6 on carbohydrate loading. Any remaining glucose will get stored as fat in adipose tissue via lipogenesis.

Carbohydrate's Role in Exercise

Carbohydrate is a primary source of energy, and the fact that glycogen is stored right in the muscle supports the importance of carbohydrate as a quick and efficient energy source for muscular contraction and movement. In fact, athletes can think of their muscles as having little gas tanks right inside of them. Just as one would not drive a car with an empty tank of gas, an athlete should be encouraged to think of "topping off" their gas tanks before exercise with carbohydrate foods and possibly during exercise as well. Aerobic exercise relies upon muscle glycogen to support ATP production. Think back to Figure 3.4 illustrating carbohydrate's contribution to energy production relative to exercise intensity. At low to moderate intensity, carbohydrate is contributing less energy *relative* to fat; however, it is still an important energy provider. The longer the exercise duration, the more likely carbohydrates stores—especially coming from muscle glycogen—become depleted. As exercise intensity increases, there is a greater reliance upon carbohydrate as an energy source. At high-intensity exercise, whether intermittent or short duration, carbohydrate is required to supply energy. Without sufficient carbohydrate availability, athletes experience increased fatigue and exercise duration or intensity or both becomes limited. Athletes want to ensure their "gas tanks" are full as they head into a training session.

Carbohydrate Recommendations

Daily Intake

Carbohydrate is an efficient energy source because it is stored directly in the muscle cell in the form of glycogen. Glycogen is also stored in the liver; this carbohydrate source can be used directly to meet the energy needs of the liver or broken down into individual glucose molecules (glycogenolysis) and released into circulation, which serves to increase or maintain blood glucose levels. During endurance exercise or inter-mittent high-intensity exercise, endogenous stores of carbohydrate can become insufficient to meet the needs of working muscle and the central nervous system (CNS), and can become the limiting factor for perfor-mance (Burke et al. 2011). Nutritional strategies to avoid carbohydrate depletion will be addressed in the following sections. These strategies are specific to before, during, or after exercise; however, the overall daily intake of carbohydrate also affects glycogen stores. Therefore, athletes need to consume adequate carbohydrate throughout the day to ensure maximal glycogen storage.

Daily carbohydrate recommendations for athletes are expressed as grams per kilogram of body weight, or g/kg. This is an absolute amount determined by body weight as compared to calculating carbohydrate intake or needs or both as a relative percentage of calories in the diet. The Dietary Reference Intakes (DRIs), which establish the dietary guidelines for nutrient intake in the United States and Canada, include Acceptable Macronutrient Distribution Ranges for the three macronutrients. Carbo-hydrates are recommended to comprise 45 to 65 percent of the caloric intake of one's diet. This is a relative term, in that it is dependent upon the total caloric intake. Forty-five to sixty-five percent of 1,600 calories will provide significantly fewer grams of carbohydrate to an athlete compared to someone who consumes 45 to 65 percent of 3,500 calories a day. So, to ensure that athletes consume sufficient carbohydrates, recommendations are based on g/kg of body weight rather than as a percentage of total caloric intake. Most athletes find that their carbohydrate needs (g/kg) will translate to 50 to 65 percent of their total caloric intake, with some endurance athletes requiring up to 70 percent of calories from carbohydrate.

In general, recommended daily intake of carbohydrate for athletes ranges from 3 to 10 g/kg of body weight, with some ultraendurance athletes needing up to 12 g/kg of body weight to ensure their glycogen stores are adequately replenished (Burke et al. 2011). See Table 4.1 for recommended daily carbohydrate intake for athletes of various sports and activities. Note that the longer the event or exercise type, or the higher the intensity of the activity, the greater the need for carbohydrate.

Table 4.1 Daily carbohydrate recommendations for athletes

Activity type	Carbohydrate recommendation (grams of carbohydrate)
Low-intensity activity or skill-based activity (includes skill work or low-intensity exercise lasting <1 hour, such as a 30-minute jog)	3–5 g/kg of body weight
Low intensity, long duration (>1 hour) Includes activities such as golf, baseball, or softball	5–7 g/kg of body weight
High intensity, short duration (1 to 30 minutes continuous) Track (200–1,500 m); short-distance cycling; rowing; figure skating; downhill skiing; swimming (100–1,500 m)	5–7 g/kg of body weight
Very high intensity, very short duration (<1 minutes) Field events (shot put, discus, high jump); track sprints (50–200 m); swimming sprints (50 m); sprint cycling (200 m); power lifting; bobsled	5–7 g/kg of body weight
Moderate intensity, moderate duration (30–60 minutes) 10K running	6–8 g/kg of body weight
Moderate to high volume or intermittent high intensity (1–3 hours) Soccer, basketball, ice hockey, lacrosse, tennis	6–10 g/kg of body weight
Moderate intensity, long duration (1+ hours) Marathon or distance running, distance swimming, Nordic skiing, distance cycling.	8–10 g/kg of body weight
Very high volume or intensity (>4–5 hours) Ultradistance running, swimming, or cycling; triathalon; adventure sports	8–12 g/kg of body weight

The recommended intakes assume individuals have an overall adequate energy (calorie) intake; individuals in an energy deficit will be discussed in Chapter 8. These carbohydrate values are ranges and should be personalized based upon individual needs. Many athletes use periodization in their training programs that include high-volume or high-intensity training along with periods of low-volume or low-intensity training. Such changes warrant adjustments in carbohydrate intake so it matches training demands.

Overall, athletes should include nutrient-dense, mostly complex carbohydrates paired with appropriate amounts of protein and fat to meet energy needs and allow for muscle recovery and growth. This dietary pattern will contribute to overall health. Athletes can strategically time the intake of the macronutrients in their diet to optimize their training and competition. Appropriate timing of carbohydrate intake can be especially helpful for optimal training and performance. When reading the following recommendations, keep in mind that specific timing recommendations of carbohydrate consumption will contribute toward an athlete's overall daily carbohydrate needs.

Timing of Intake

Carbohydrate Recommendations Before Exercise

Numerous research studies have supported the performance benefits of consuming adequate preexercise carbohydrate (Ormsbee, Bach, and Baur 2014). Nutrition strategies that focus on optimizing glycogen stores, or "topping off" the gas tanks, ensure an adequate fuel supply to working muscle. Total body glycogen stores can typically be normalized within a 24-hour period (Burke et al. 2011), although overnight, liver glycogen stores can be depleted by up to 80 percent. Much of the overnight depletion comes from liver glycogen, with muscle glycogen stores experiencing minimal impact (Ormsbee, Bach, and Baur 2014). The period leading up to exercise—that is, up to 4 hours—can be vital to ensure adequate muscle and liver glycogen.

It is recommended that athletes engaging in endurance or intense exercise, or high-volume resistance exercise, consume 1 to 4 g of carbohydrate per kilogram of body weight (g/kg) 1 to 4 hours before exercise commences. That is, athletes should consume 1 g/kg/body weight 1 hour before exercise, 2 g/kg/body weight 2 hours before exercise, 3 g/kg/body weight 3 hours before exercise, or 4 g/kg/body weight 4 hours before exercise. Research does not show differences in performance when carbohydrate is consumed at different points within this window (4 hours before, for example, versus 1 hour before) as long as the appropriate amount is consumed according to the time before exercise. So, practicalities of eating as well as the ability to tolerate food before exercise may dictate when is best to eat. Some athletes can consume a moderate meal containing carbohydrate an hour before exercise; most individuals, however, find it best to give themselves 2 to 4 hours for their pre-event meal to allow for digestion to occur. As long as they are consuming adequate amounts of carbohydrate (1 to 4 g) within 1 to 4 hours, they should have sufficient glycogen stores.

Consuming carbohydrates causes an increase in blood glucose, which, in turn, causes the pancreas to release insulin into the blood. One to four hours is probably sufficient time for blood glucose and insulin levels to return to normal; however, less than 1 hour may not be. Eating less than an hour prior to exercise can be problematic for some individuals. In addition to GI distress, some athletes can have adverse drops in blood glucose related to the increase in insulin levels resulting from the recent consumption of carbohydrate-containing foods. Exercise also initiates an insulin-independent mechanism of clearing glucose out of the blood and into the cell by increasing GLUT4 translocation. The net effect of increased insulin levels *and* exercise-induced GLUT4 translocation is that glucose can be cleared out of the blood too quickly and can result in exercise-induced hypoglycemia. While these perturbations in blood glucose levels are transient and return to normal within about 20 minutes, athletes can feel shaky, queasy, and light-headed in the meantime. To avoid this negative reaction it is important to allow 1 hour or more for digestion of carbohydrate-containing foods prior to exercise in individuals experiencing these symptoms (Ormsbee, Bach, and Baur 2014).

While glycemic index may have limited utility for athletes overall, one exception is that it may help diminish the likelihood of exercise-induced hypoglycemia. The glycemic index measures the blood glucose response to carbohydrate-containing foods and consuming low glycemic index carbohydrates may result in an attenuated blood insulin and glucose response. Because blood glucose levels do not rapidly increase after eating a low-glycemic index food, less insulin is released and exercise-induced hypoglycemia is less likely. Ingesting CHO prior to exercise has also been shown to suppress fatty acid oxidation, but some research suggests that choosing low-glycemic index foods limits the effect. However, carbohydrate that is consumed *during* exercise will impact blood glucose levels as well as fuel substrate utilization, thus minimizing the effects of the glycemic characteristics of the pre-event food (Burke et al. 2011). This indicates that selecting low-glycemic index foods prior to exercise in efforts to affect metabolism and substrate utilization during exercise is only effective if carbohydrate is not consumed during exercise. Research on this topic is equivocal in that some studies report an endurance performance benefit of selecting low-glycemic index foods, but most do not. Based on the available research, strategies that focus on using the glycemic index to consume low-glycemic index foods prior to exercise may best suited for individuals who do not consume carbohydrate during an event or those who are more susceptible to exercise-induced hypoglycemia, since at the very least there does not appear to be a disadvantage of consuming low glycemic index foods (Burke 2010; Ormsbee, Bach, and Baur 2014). More research is needed to provide generalized recommendations regarding glycemic index.

Carbohydrate Recommendations During Exercise

Substantial evidence supports the benefit of consuming carbohydrate during exercise of specified duration and intensity. Interestingly, this benefit is realized through multiple mechanisms in the body.

Historically, research looking at carbohydrate intake during exercise has been based on the assumption that consuming carbohydrate increases glucose availability, allowing athletes to maintain an exercise intensity for a longer duration, which ultimately may result in enhanced performance. While there is validity to this statement, recent research has identified independent mechanisms by which carbohydrate impacts performance. For exercise lasting more than 2 hours, exogenous carbohydrate provision prevents hypoglycemia, supports carbohydrate oxidation, and thus allows athletes to exercise longer or harder or both (Jeukendrup 2014).

However, when carbohydrate is provided during exercise shorter than 2 hours, it is not the increased glucose availability that seems to enhance performance since muscle glycogen stores are not the limiting factor. Rather, the effect is seen on the CNS. Specifically, when carbohydrate-containing foods are consumed, receptors in the mouth sense the presence of carbohydrate, resulting in a sense of well-being that allows the athlete to train harder (Burke et al. 2011). This is supported by research that demonstrates improved performance with administration of a carbohydrate-containing mouth rinse versus a placebo (Jeukendrup 2014) where carbohydrate is not actually consumed, but its presence is merely sensed in the mouth. While the exact mechanisms are not fully understood, research has clearly shown a performance benefit at shorter-duration, higher-intensity exercise (about 1 hour) when carbohydrate is detected in the mouth but is not necessarily digested (Jeukendrup 2014).

The recommended amount of carbohydrate to be consumed during exercise depends upon duration and intensity. For exercise lasting 45 to 75 minutes, only small amounts of carbohydrate are needed and even a mouth rinse with carbohydrate is sufficient (see Table 4.2); the exception would be if an athletes has not eaten for 5 to 6 hours. In this case, their need for carbohydrate can be as great as 30 to 60 g/hr. For exercise lasting 1 to 2 hours, 30 g/hr supports optimal performance. At longer-duration exercise, exogenous carbohydrate becomes an important energy source and there seems to be a dose-dependent relationship. With exercise

Table 4.2 *Carbohydrate recommendations during exercise*

Duration of exercise	Amount of carbohydrate needed	Recommended type of carbohydrate
30–75 minutes	Small amounts (<30 g) or mouth rinse	Single or multiple transportable carbohydrate
1–2 hours	30 g/hr	Single or multiple transportable carbohydrate
2–3 hours	30–60 g/hr	Single or multiple transportable carbohydrate
>2.5 hours	60–90 g/hr	Only multiple transportable carbohydrates

lasting longer than 2 hours, a carbohydrate intake of 60 to 90 g/hr seems to result in peak performance (Jeukendrup 2014).

Keep in mind that exercise intensity is still an important consideration. Tour de France cyclists riding for many hours at high intensities are oxidizing glucose at high rates and thus should be consuming the upper end of the range. The 5-hour marathon runner may be exercising at a more moderate intensity and with this lower oxidation rate may only need 60 g/hr, for example. See Table 4.3 for a list of the carbohydrate content of common foods consumed during exercise.

The type of carbohydrate may have significant implications as well. The previous belief that maximal carbohydrate oxidation rate was 60 g/hr was based upon research investigating glucose. This is because glucose metabolism is limited by intestinal absorption of glucose. Glucose relies

Table 4.3 Carbohydrate content of foods consumed during exercise

Food	Amount	Carbohydrate (g)
Gatorade™ Original or Endurance	8 oz	14
Gatorade Prime Energy Chews	6 chews	24
Powerade™ Sports Drink	8 oz	14–15 (depending upon flavor)
Hammer™ Heed	1 scoop/1 svg	27
Hammer Perpetuem	2 scoops/1 svg	54
Clif™ Bars	1 bar	41–45
Clif Shot Gel	1 packet	22–24
Clif Shot Blocks	3 blocks	23–24
PowerBar™ Bar	1 bar	43–45
PowerBar Energy Wafers	1 package	29–31
Honey Stinger™ Energy Gel	1 packet	24–27
Honey Stinger Waffle	1 waffle	21
Sport Beans™	1 packet	25
Banana	1 large banana	27
Red roasted potato	1 medium	29
Fig newton	2 cookies	22
Peanut butter and jelly	1 sandwich	39–54 (depends upon bread and jelly amount)

Note: Information obtained from manufacturers' websites.

upon sodium-dependent transporter (SGLT1) for absorption and this becomes saturated when carbohydrate intake reaches 60 g/hr (Jeukendrup 2014). To address this limitation, it has been suggested to include fructose. Fructose has its own transporter and can be absorbed through a different pathway. While consuming fructose alone may cause GI distress, consuming glucose plus fructose seems to result in less (GI) distress, which can permit greater exercise capacity. Thus, choosing a mix of carbohydrates, such as glucose and fructose, that can be transported across the intestinal wall by multiple transports results in greater carbohydrate oxidation and allows carbohydrate intake during exercise to reach 90 g/hr without GI distress (Wilson, Rhodes, and Ingraham 2015). For exercise lasting 2.5 hours or longer, exogenous carbohydrate sources are especially important for maintaining power output. This is why many sport nutrition products are now formulated to include both glucose and fructose, providing an accessible medium for these nutrients.

Whether the carbohydrates are in liquid form or solid form seem to have similar performance-enhancing effects, so one is not necessarily advantageous over another in regard to performance. This allows athletes to choose that which is preferable or more practical or both. Some athletes find sport nutrition drinks, or sports drinks (such as Gatorade, Powerade, or homemade varieties), to be efficient in meeting their needs given that sports drinks provide all the essential nutrients—carbohydrates, electrolytes, and fluids. The ideal carbohydrate concentration of sports drinks is 6 to 8 percent. This allows for adequate carbohydrate intake compared to a less concentrated formula, but is not too concentrated so that it would cause GI distress.

Most commercial formulas are within this range, though they vary slightly. Gatorade is at the lower end of the range with 6 percent carbohydrate concentration, whereas Powerade is at the higher end of the range at about 8 percent. The higher percentage will deliver more glucose to working muscles, but tolerance may decrease as the concentration increases. Athletes should try different products and see what works best for them. Some athletes choose to get carbohydrates from a combination of carbohydrate-containing beverages and from food sources, while other athletes choose to drink water and obtain their carbohydrates (and electrolytes when needed) from foods. These are all acceptable approaches and just depend upon preference. The key is to ensure all needs are being met in accordance with the demands of the activity.

There are athletes who believe they cannot tolerate food or that they cannot even drink water during exercise. These athletes should understand that depending upon the duration, intensity, and frequency of exercise, inadequate provision of appropriate nutrients becomes a limiting factor during exercise. Not only is performance impaired, but an athlete's mood and psychological well-being during exercise suffers due to carbohydrate's effect on CNS. Dehydration and inadequate fuel can make exercise feel more strenuous and tiresome, impairing an athlete's ability to train hard. In working with a sports dietitian or nutrition expert these athletes can be coached on how to "train" their bodies to tolerate nutrients needed for training. Through consistent and gradual exposure to essential nutrients, tolerance of foods and fluids can improve. These efforts should begin well before competition so that not only can they enhance their training, but also by race day these athletes have optimized their nutrition plan.

Some athletes successfully meet their exercise nutrient needs with sport nutrition products. Other athletes desire to take a more "whole foods" approach in efforts to minimize or limit intake of processed foods. Some athletes use a combination of tactics. All approaches can provide adequate nutrients if the recommendations are followed regarding fluid, carbohydrate, and electrolyte requirements. For example, some cyclists consume peanut butter and jelly sandwiches, mashed sweet potatoes, and homemade sports drinks to meet their hourly nutrient needs; others consume sports gels and sport drinks to achieve the same goal. Some endurance runners use salted, boiled potatoes in combinations with fig cookies and sports gels. There are a variety of food and fluid options for athletes to consume during exercise that can be selected according to convenience, preference, and personal nutrition philosophy.

Of note is that the majority of studies examining the effects of carbohydrate during exercise have been conducted on cyclists and runners. Less research is available on team sports involving intermittent, high-intensity effort such as soccer or football. It is believed that the recommendations are similar to those of endurance sports, though the timing of carbohydrate consumption should be based on the sport type and other practical considerations (Beelen, Cermak, and van Loon 2015). For example, in a team sport such as soccer or rugby, athletes may be limited to consumption of carbohydrate during half-time due to lack of access to foods and beverages during playing time. Additionally, there is some research indicating carbohydrate consumption during sport can improve reaction time, concentration, and power in various team sports and in skiing events. It is important that athletes keep in mind carbohydrate's role in CNS functioning as well as its importance for muscular contraction to emphasize its importance for skill-based work.

Carbohydrate Recommendations After Exercise

Many athletes realize the value of protein consumption postworkout; but often underappreciated, however, is the importance of consuming adequate carbohydrate at this time as well. Short-duration, intense exercise can significantly lower muscle glycogen stores, and exhaustive endurance exercise can result in near depletion (Beelen et al. 2010). Because of the potential performance impairment of exercising with low glycogen stores, as well as the associated fatigue, it is important that athletes replete their stores to optimize their training capacity.

There are two distinct phases of muscle glycogen synthesis postexercise. The first phase is characterized by rapid glycogen synthesis within the first 30 to 60 minutes, and operates independent of insulin. As described previously, exercise stimulates the translocation of the glucose transporter GLUT4 to the cell membrane and causes blood glucose to be taken up into the cell. This GLUT4 translocation, as well as the large concentration gradient of high glucose outside of the cell to low glucose inside of the cell, is responsible for the increased rate of glycogen synthesis in this first phase. This initial, rapid phase of glycogen synthesis only occurs in the presence of very low glycogen stores (such as the result of exhaustive exercise), when stores are 25 percent or lower than baseline levels (Price et al. 1994). While the rate of synthesis can be very high in this phase, if glucose is not available in sufficient quantities in the blood, resynthesis will quickly stall out in an effort to maintain blood glucose levels.

The second phase of muscle glycogen synthesis is insulin-dependent. The rate of synthesis is not as rapid as in the initial phase, though the second phase is still an important stimulator of muscle glycogen synthesis and is not reliant upon severe depletion of glycogen stores. Exercise increases the cell's sensitivity to insulin, and so postexercise glucose uptake and glycogen synthesis are increased (Beelen et al. 2010). Thus, nutrition intervention that enhances the effects of insulin, such as eating carbohydrate-containing foods, is essential during this second phase of muscle glycogen synthesis.

Both phases of glycogen synthesis are reliant upon provision of adequate dietary carbohydrate postexercise. Various amounts of carbohydrate have been studied, and research indicates that consuming 1.2 g of carbohydrate per kilogram of body weight per hour (1.2 g/kg/hr) up to several hours after exercise seems to be the optimal amount to maximize muscle glycogen synthesis (Poole et al. 2010). Total synthesis can be optimized when carbohydrate is provided over several small-to-moderate feedings at regular intervals, versus consuming one large carbohydrate meal in the same time frame. For example, an athlete can consume a carbohydrate snack every 15 to 30 minutes for up to 4 hours that amounts to 1.2 g/kg/hr for optimal glycogen synthesis.

However, consuming this amount is not always feasible for athletes due to logistic or practical constraints or both. Coingestion of protein with carbohydrate has been shown to be beneficial for muscle glycogen resynthesis and may decrease the amount of carbohydrate needed. Protein ingestion stimulates insulin release and research indicates that when carbohydrate intake is suboptimal postexercise (<1.0 g/kg/hr), coingestion of protein and amino acids (~0.4 g/kg/hr) can support maximal glycogen synthesis; however, no additional benefit was seen when carbohydrate intake was optimal (1.2 g/kg/hr). While additional functions of protein and protein resynthesis will be discussed in the next section, protein does help athletes maximize muscle glycogen resynthesis when postexercise carbohydrate intake is less than optimal. Additionally, there are advantages for the athlete looking to lose or maintain body weight by consuming slightly less carbohydrate in the presence of adequate protein, which will be discussed in Chapter 8.

Timing of carbohydrate consumption is an important consideration. The aforementioned recommendations are provided for maximal muscle glycogen synthesis at a rapid rate. This maximal glycogen synthesis rate is especially important in situations when athletes have less than 8 hours before their next workout, such as in the case of two-a-day practices or tournament-style competitions. However, the timing of carbohydrate intake appears to be less important when there are 24 hours to recover before the next exercise bout. In these situations, it is more about the total carbohydrate intake over the course of 24 hours versus the intake immediately after and up to 4 hours after exercise. Knowing an athlete's exercise and competition schedule is essential for determining optimal recovery nutrition strategies.

Similar recommendations apply to the type of carbohydrate intake postexercise; if there are less than 8 hours between exercise bouts, the type of carbohydrate may be important. It appears that high glycemic index foods may promote faster glycogen synthesis rates (Poole et al. 2010) than low glycemic index foods. However, when athletes have more than 8 hours to recover, the type of carbohydrate may be less important. It also appears that liquid form versus solid food form does not affect muscle glycogen synthesis, though there are other practical considerations that will be discussed at the end of the section in "Putting it all together."

Protein

Protein is a popular macronutrient among athletes. In fact, many athletes believe they need to consume large amounts of dietary protein to perform well. Understanding the structure and function of protein, as well as its metabolism in the body is essential to educating athletes on the truths, and myths, of protein requirements for athletic performance.

Structure, Basic Function, and Food Forms

Protein is composed of carbon, hydrogen, and oxygen, but unlike fat and carbohydrate, protein also contains nitrogen. Protein is composed of at least one or more long chain of amino acids, and these individual amino acids, along with the protein's structure, determine the protein's function. There are 20 different amino acids that make up proteins. Amino acids are typically classified according to their essentiality or nonessentiality; that is, nonessential amino acids, referred to as dispensable amino acids, are those that can be synthesized by the liver. Essential, or indispensable amino acids, are those the body must obtain from food sources because it cannot make these amino acids on its own. Conditionally indispensable amino acids are those that the body can synthesize under normal, healthy conditions, but due to disease state or nutrient deficiency the body must obtain these amino acids from the diet. See Table 4.4.

Protein can be classified according to its quality, that is, its content and proportionality of indispensable amino acids. A high-quality, or complete, protein contains all the indispensable amino acids in the amounts needed by humans. Food sources of complete proteins include eggs, milk, yogurt, meat, fish, poultry, and soy. Incomplete proteins are those that do not contain sufficient amounts of indispensable amino acids. Incomplete proteins are found in plant foods such as grains, legumes, and vegetables. A diet containing only incomplete protein sources, if consumed in insufficient quantities, may not provide adequate amounts of indispensable amino acids, which may impair the body's ability to make certain proteins required for health, recovery, and muscle growth.

Contrary to popular belief, most plant-based proteins do contain all of the essential amino acids (EAA); however, their amino acid profile often falls short of that of the reference protein (albumin). Thus they are considered lower quality. Nonetheless, since individuals rarely consume single food items at a meal or even over the course of the day, assuming the individual is consuming a variety of plant-based proteins and consuming

Table 4.4 *Dispensable, indispensable, and conditionally indispensable amino acids*

Dispensable	Indispensable	Conditionally indispensable
Alanine	Histidine	Arginine
Aspartic acid	Isoleucine	Cysteine
Asparagine	Leucine	Glutamine
Glutamic acid	Lysine	Glycine
Serine	Methionine	Proline
	Phenylalanine	Tyrosine
	Threonine	
	Tryptophan	
	Valine	

enough total protein, meeting amino acid requirements will not be difficult. Additionally, by pairing certain plant-based protein foods, known as complimentary proteins, the amino acids profile becomes complete and provides adequate amounts of all of the indispensable amino acids. For example, legumes that are low in tryptophan and methionine can be paired with grains containing greater amounts of these amino acids; the isoleucine and lysine found in legumes complement the low content of these amino acids in grains. Rice and beans, peanut butter and whole wheat (bread), and hummus with pita bread are all examples of complementary proteins. These foods do not need to be paired together in the same meal but rather consumed throughout the day.

Protein has many functions in the human body. Proteins serve as catalysts in the form of enzymes, and support immune function as immunoglobulins. Proteins act as chemical messengers in the form of hormones, and provide a structural role in contractile proteins and collagen. Proteins help transport nutrients and other substances throughout the body such as albumin and lipoproteins. Proteins function as both an intra- and extracellular buffer. This is not even an exhaustive list, as proteins serve many other functions. However, especially as it pertains to athletes, proteins are essential for maintaining fluid balance, and they serve as a structural component of bone and connective tissue, and help repair tissue damage and build muscle. So, while many athletes often know of protein's role in muscle protein synthesis, it is important they understand protein's diverse functions in the body.

Categorizing the various sources of protein into plant and animal sources can be helpful when making food choices. Animal sources of protein include meat, fish, and poultry; eggs; and dairy. Plant foods that provide contributable amounts of protein are legumes that include soy and soy products, nuts and seeds, and whole grains. Athletes should understand that different types of protein come in different packages and thus offer diverse nutritional benefits. For example, an animal source of protein such as chicken will provide protein as well as iron, vitamin B_{12}, and zinc. Kidney beans, on the other hand, contain protein, but they also provide potassium, magnesium, and folate.

It is a misconception that animal protein sources are "superior" to plant proteins. As mentioned previously, complementary proteins can be combined to provide the indispensable amino acids that athletes need. While the digestibility and thus bioavailability is greater in animal protein sources, vegetarian athletes can still meet their protein needs through careful menu planning. Considerations for vegetarian athletes will be addressed in Chapter 8. Athletes who are not vegetarian should not rely exclusively upon animal protein foods, but rather should include diverse plant and animal protein sources to ensure a wide variety of nutrients obtained from these foods.

Protein Metabolism

When protein is consumed from food sources, the protein is digested into its individual amino acids through the enzymatic action of proteases. Individual amino acids then become part of the amino acid pool as do the amino acids from the catabolism of body tissue. Since the body cannot store amino acids or proteins, there is constant protein turnover in the body. Some proteins are continually being synthesized, while others are being digested. If the rate of synthesis equals the rate of catabolism, there is protein balance. If the rate of protein breakdown exceeds the rate of protein synthesis, one is in negative protein balance, or a state of catabolism. This happens in periods of illness, inadequate physical activity, or when dietary intake of protein is insufficient.

Protein's Role in Exercise

Many athletes are seeking to achieve **muscle hypertrophy**. For muscle mass to increase, a positive protein balance must be achieved whereby the rate of muscle protein synthesis exceeds that of muscle protein breakdown. While dietary consumption of protein can stimulate muscle protein synthesis, to actually have a positive net balance that results in muscle hypertrophy, there also needs to be a loading stimulus to skeletal muscle. This requires resistance exercise. Thus, consuming protein in the diet alone is insufficient to increase muscle mass. Similarly, engaging in resistance exercise in the absence of dietary protein intake will not only be insufficient to increase muscle mass, but may also result in a negative muscle protein balance, that is, the muscle is in a catabolic state (Tipton and Sharp 2005). Therefore, resistance exercise in the presence of **hyper-aminoacidemia**, or having excess amino acids in the blood, is required to stimulate muscle protein synthesis. The timing of protein intake is also important, and this will be discussed in the following section on "Protein Recommendations."

Another misconception is that protein is a good source of energy for exercise. In reality, the body prefers to use carbohydrate and fat as an energy source because they are more efficiently utilized by muscle cells. Using protein as an energy source is very inefficient, in that the process of converting protein into energy actually consumes energy before energy can be produced. This is because the amino group must be removed from the amino acid through deamination or transamination and a then carbon skeleton, or α–keto acid, is formed. These carbon skeletons can then be metabolized to produce energy, that is, glucose via **gluconeogenesis**, ketone bodies, or other substances. However, these pathways require the input of energy before energy can be produced. The net yield of glucose from protein metabolism is significantly less than is the amount of glucose produced from carbohydrates via glycolysis. The result is that protein is a very inefficient energy source.

Additionally, the body prefers to utilize amino acids for anabolic purposes. Think of the many functions of protein in the body. Amino acids resulting from protein metabolism are needed for muscle and tissue synthesis, for bone turnover, and for the production of other body proteins, among other functions. Thus, adequate carbohydrate and, to some degree, fat help to "spare" protein from being metabolized for energy production and to maintain energy balance. Under normal circumstances, protein contributes only ~5 percent of energy; under periods of starvation or during prolonged periods of exercise, where there is insufficient carbohydrate availability, this amount may increase up to 18 percent of energy contribution. This is not a desired nutritional status and dietary strategies can help prevent excessive protein oxidation.

Protein Recommendations

Protein is a macronutrient often misunderstood among the athletic population and there are also misconceptions as to the optimal amount of protein needed by athletes for muscle tissue repair and growth. Protein does much more than build muscle; rather, it has many essential functions in the body. Yet, contrary to what some athletes believe, protein is not an efficient or optimal fuel source. The following is a review of the most current research regarding optimal protein intake for athletes.

Daily Intake

The daily recommended protein intake for athletes is an area of research that is not without controversy. There is consensus that athletes have increased protein needs above those of sedentary individuals, though specific amounts are disputed. Part of the uncertainty is based upon methodological limitations when studying protein needs, and some confusion comes from defining what an athlete "needs" versus what is considered optimal intake. Providing appropriate protein recommendations for athletes requires an understanding of these issues.

As part of the DRIs, the Recommended Dietary Allowance (RDA) for protein in the United States and Canada for nonathletic adults is 0.8 grams per kilogram of body weight (0.8 g/kg). However, this is not necessarily an amount that an individual *should* be consuming, but rather is the amount needed to avoid the negative consequences of protein deficiency in 98 percent of the healthy population. Even with nonathletic populations, some researchers and professionals believe higher intakes would be beneficial. However, given that the AMDR for protein is 10 to 35 percent of one's total caloric intake, this wide range can allow for higher protein intakes and still be considered "acceptable."

Protein recommendations for athletic and nonathletic populations are typically based upon nitrogen balance studies that try to assess total body protein metabolism. The process measures nitrogen intake (by looking at protein intake from food records, since protein is the only source of dietary nitrogen) and nitrogen excretion in the urine. Positive nitrogen balance occurs during periods of growth and repair and indicates an increase in total body protein. Negative nitrogen balance occurs during periods of illness, burns, injury, and fasting when nitrogen excretion exceeds that of consumption and total body protein stores are being diminished. Nitrogen balance occurs when nitrogen intake equals the rate of nitrogen excretion and indicates that protein needs are being met. Nitrogen balance studies have become a method frequently employed to assess protein status within populations.

One challenge, however, is that using nitrogen balance as an indicator of protein adequacy does not translate well to athletes. There are numerous methodological concerns with using nitrogen balance studies as a basis for protein recommendations. Further, the goal of the RDA is to prevent deficiencies by replacing losses. This does not equate to what is optimal or desirable for athletes. Athletes are not merely trying to prevent deficiency; rather, athletes are typically striving for positive adaptations from training. These adaptations include repairing and replacing damaged proteins, remodeling protein, supporting training-induced adaptations in metabolic functioning, contributing to lean muscle mass accrual, and enhancing immune functioning (Phillips 2012).

With this in mind, research has set out to better determine what a truly optimal intake of protein is for athletes. The recommended daily intake for athletes falls in the range of 1.2 to 1.7 g/kg/day though can be as high as 2.0 g/kg/day such as with athletes with weight management goals, as will be discussed in Chapter 8. Resistance athletes benefit from higher protein recommendations because protein, and specifically the EAAs (see Table 4.4) derived from protein, are what stimulate muscle protein synthesis and inhibit muscle protein breakdown. Endurance exercise also stimulates muscle protein synthesis, though to a smaller extent than resistance exercise. Additionally, consumption of dietary protein may preserve lean muscle mass. Prolonged exercise results in increased amino acid oxidation for energy production. This includes long-duration endurance exercise (over 3 hours) that relies upon the oxidation of leucine, a branched-chain amino acid found in certain protein sources, for additional energy substrate. Consumption of exogenous protein sources can minimize the breakdown of muscle tissue for the oxidation of amino acids. Finally, after resistance and endurance training, adequate protein consumption supplies amino acids for tissue repair. See Table 4.5 outlining the recommended daily protein intake for athletes.

Table 4.5 Recommended daily protein intake for individuals

Level of activity	Recommended daily protein intake
Sedentary adults	0.8 g/kg
Recreational athletes	1.0 g/kg
Endurance athletes	1.2–1.4 g/kg
Ultraendurance athletes	1.2–1.7 g/kg
Strength athletes	1.2–1.7 g/kg

Can Athletes Consume Too Much Protein?

Protein intake among athletes tends to be adequate if not higher than the recommended amounts for athletes. For example, strength athletes may consume 2.0 to 2.5 g/kg/day with some athletes reaching up to 3.5 g/kg/day (Tarnopolsky 2004). Endurance athletes typically consume the recommended amount of 1.2 to 1.6 g/kg, though some female endurance athletes report lower intakes (Phillips 2004). While there does not seem to be an added benefit of eating more than the recommended 1.2 to 1.7 g/kg/day, there is the question if there is potential for harm.

A common perception is that a high protein intake would stress the kidneys and potentially result in kidney damage; however, in individuals with healthy renal functioning, this does not appear to be the case. There is also a question as to whether or not a high protein intake would have a detrimental impact on bone health such that it would decrease bone mineral density, though there is little support for this as well. In fact, recent research has shown that a protein intake at the higher end of the recommended range seems have an anabolic effect on bone through its stimulation of the hormone IGF-1 (Remer, Krupp, and Shi 2014).

What is of concern with an excess protein intake among athletes is its impact on overall dietary intake. If an athlete consumes excess dietary protein in the presence of adequate carbohydrate and fat, this could result in excess caloric consumption leading to excess weight gain. Some athletes believe whatever protein they do not use, they will excrete in their urine. On the contrary, excess protein (just like excess fat or excess carbohydrate) gets stored as fat when intake is above energy needs. Thus, to remain in energy balance and still consume higher amounts of protein, athletes would have to decrease their fat or carbohydrate or both intake. Inadequate fat intake may result in an inadequate intake of essential fatty acids along with other health concerns. Consuming insufficient carbohydrates not only has potential health effects, including micronutrient and fiber deficiencies, but can also be detrimental to performance, as previously discussed. Even high-intensity, short-duration exercise that is common to strength athletes relies upon carbohydrate as an essential fuel source. Consuming too much dietary protein at the expense of adequate carbohydrate intake may have serious effects on performance.

Timing of Intake

Protein Recommendations Before and During Exercise

The potential benefit of consuming protein before and during exercise depends in part on the exercise type. In 2001, a study by Tipton et al. found that ingestion of 6 g of EAAs and 35 g of sucrose ingested prior to exercise increased muscle protein synthesis postexercise more than when the mixture was consumed immediately after exercise (Tipton et al. 2001). Since that time, research has generally, though not unequivocally, supported the benefit of consuming some EAAs before resistance training to increase muscle protein synthesis. The same has not been found for endurance exercise. There does not seem to be a performance benefit when protein is consumed during endurance exercise, given that carbohydrate intake is sufficient, thought there is some research indicating that protein intake during ultraendurance exercise (>3 hours) may attenuate muscle protein breakdown, as well as improve skeletal muscle reconditioning (van Loon 2014). Thus consuming small-to-moderate amounts of protein during ultraendurance events may have a beneficial effect.

To summarize, strength athletes may find benefit to add some protein before or during their workout, though the consensus is that postexercise consumption of protein has the most beneficial effect. Ultraendurance athletes may also benefit from consuming some protein during their exercise though adequate carbohydrate intake is of utmost importance.

Protein Recommendations After Exercise

The hormonal environment postexercise is considered anabolic in that it promotes muscle protein synthesis, and this requires adequate substrate availability. The effect of carbohydrate and protein on insulin secretion has already been discussed in relation to this enhanced hormonal environment. However, adequate protein intake postexercise also plays a crucial role in repairing or rebuilding muscle proteins that have been damaged from exercise, as well as stimulating muscle mass accrual.

The optimal amount of protein postexercise has been studied extensively and it appears that 20 to 25 g of high-quality protein maximizes muscle protein synthesis; there is no additional benefit of protein intakes greater than this amount (Phillips 2012). High-quality protein is characterized here by its EAA profile. Approximately 10 g of EAA maximizes muscle protein synthesis, which translates to about 20 to 25 g of high intact protein sources. This includes eggs, dairy, or lean meats. Soy is also a good source of EAAs, though its content of leucine, a major stimulator of muscle protein synthesis, is less than that of animal protein sources. The anabolic environment is highest immediately after exercise, though this window extends for up to 2 hours postexercise. Ideally, protein consumption occurs as soon as possible upon completion of exercise regardless of whether these nutrients are consumed from food sources or from beverages as long as total consumption is adequate.

One challenge faced by many athletes is that after exercising they report their appetite is blunted and this can impede sufficient intake of nutrients. The hormonal milieu resulting from exercise is partially to blame for this effect. Decreased appetite seems to peak immediately postexercise, and yet this is a time when consumption of protein can optimize protein synthesis. Taking advantage of this anabolic window is often desired. One solution found to be helpful is to consume beverages containing the necessary nutrients. Drinking liquids when hunger is blunted can be less offensive than trying to eat solid foods. This strategy has resulted in the popularity of recovery beverages. Protein shakes, for example, are quite prevalent, especially among, but not limited to, strength athletes. These drinks can be appropriate if there is adequate carbohydrate, there is not an excessive amount of protein, and the right types of protein are included. Protein supplements are discussed in more detail in Chapter 7.

One study attempted to ascertain the optimal recovery beverage to meet the needs of athletes after an exhaustive workout. The researchers' conclusion was that consuming chocolate milk was indeed an optimal recovery strategy (Spaccarotella and Andzel 2011). Milk has potassium and sodium, which assist in electrolyte replacement. Milk contains whey, a fast-acting protein that attenuates muscle protein breakdown, and casein, a slow-acting protein that promotes muscle protein synthesis. Milk also has a desirable profile of branched-chain amino acids, leucine, isoleucine, and valine, which are known to slow muscle breakdown and stimulate muscle protein synthesis, particularly leucine. The addition of chocolate contributes greater carbohydrate to glycogen synthesis. Of course, chocolate milk is not the only option, but it is a convenient, effective, and inexpensive strategy for many athletes. Chocolate soymilk can be an option for individuals with lactose intolerance, though the amino acid and protein profile of soymilk is not quite as desirable as that of dairy milk.

Lipids

Structure, Basic Functions, and Food Forms

Lipids are a macronutrient providing energy and other essential nutrients to the body. Lipids are composed of carbon (C), hydrogen (H), and oxygen (O) similar to carbohydrate. Lipids are the most energy dense of the macronutrients and provide 9 kcal/kg, versus the four calories in 1 g of carbohydrate and protein. Lipids are also anhydrous, meaning they do not store water with them, whereas for every gram of glycogen that is stored 3 g of water are stored with it. We would weigh a lot more if we stored all of our energy as glycogen. These characteristics make lipids a very efficient storage form of energy.

Triglycerides are the main form of lipid consumed in the diet. Triglycerides are composed of three fatty acids, or chains of carbon and hydrogen atoms with a carboxyl group at one end and a methyl group at the other, and a "backbone" glycerol molecule that is attached via an ester bond (see Figure 4.1).

Glycerol   3 Fatty acid chains

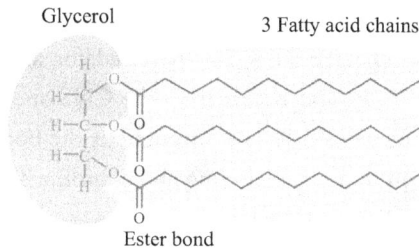

Ester bond

Figure 4.1 A Triglyceride

Dietary triglycerides (or dietary fats) are classified as either saturated or unsaturated (mono or poly). In reality, individual fatty acid chains may be fully saturated with hydrogen atoms (saturated fats), may have one double bond between carbon atoms (monounsaturated fatty acid), or may have two or more carbon-to-carbon double bonds (polyunsaturated fatty acids). As a consequence, the dietary triglyceride (or fat) is categorized based on the chemical structure of the majority of fatty acids. For example, olive oil is considered to be a monounsaturated fat, but it contains 8 percent polyunsaturated fatty acids and 13 percent saturated fatty acids. In general terms, saturated fats are typically solid at room temperature; butter and the white marbling in meats are considered to be primarily made up of saturated fatty acids. Saturated fats are also found in tropical oils such as coconut, palm, and palm kern oil but these tend to be liquid at room temperature. Unsaturated fats are usually liquid at room temperature. Monounsaturated fats are found in foods such as almonds, avocado, and olive oil. Food sources of polyunsaturated fats include vegetable oils such as soybean and corn oil, and fatty fish such as salmon and tuna fish. Trans fats are unsaturated fats that are naturally occurring in very small amounts, but primarily are consumed from products containing artificially derived trans fats. These fats have been chemically modified to be more shelf stable by making the *cis* configuration of the double bond a *trans* configuration. Trans fats are found in commercial baked goods, some fast food products, coffee creamers, and snacks foods and should be avoided.

While a primary function of fat is to provide energy at rest and during low- to moderate-intensity exercise, fat has many roles in the body. Body fat acts as storage vessel of energy during times of famine and as an insulator to help maintain body temperature, as well as surround and protect vital organs. Dietary fat is also required for absorption of fat-soluble vitamins A, D, E, and K. Fat lines the CNS and plays a role in signal transduction between cells and throughout the body. Fat is also a precursor to other compounds, including cholesterol, which is important for cell membranes, vitamin D synthesis, and the synthesis of important hormones.

Fat Metabolism

When triglycerides are consumed from foods, they are broken down in the small intestine through bile emulsification and hydrolyzed predominantly through pancreatic enzymes to yield free fatty acids. Short- and medium-chain fatty acids go through the portal vein and enter into circulation where they bind with a carrier protein such as albumin. Long-chain fatty acids are resynthesized into triglycerides and are packaged into lipoproteins called chylomicrons in the mucosal cells of the small intestine. These chylomicrons slowly enter into circulation via lymphatic vessels. The chylomicron, now in the blood, eventually comes into contact with an enzyme called lipoprotein lipase. This enzyme is found on the walls of capillaries that innervate muscle and fat cells and causes the fatty acids within the triglyceride portion of the chylomicron to be released and is rapidly absorbed by muscle and fat cells. Once inside the cell, the free fatty acids will either be used as a substrate for energy via aerobic metabolism or be repackaged once again and stored as adipose or intramuscular triglycerides. The fact that muscle can store triglycerides is significant, just as they can store carbohydrates. These proximal storage forms allow for accessible energy provision.

Fat's Role in Exercise

Just as some carbohydrates have healthier properties than others, not all fats are created equally. Avoiding fat altogether is not recommended and a low-fat diet can be a detriment to performance as well as health. However, type of fats included in the diet is of importance. Trans fat should be limited or avoided in the diet as high intakes of these types of fats increase ones risk for heart disease (Ackland et al. 2012; Eckel et al. 2014), and there is no need for trans fat in the diet. Currently, there are efforts being made to ban the use of trans fats in food manufacturing, though the outcome is yet to be seen.

There is evidence to support that limiting dietary saturated fat intake may decrease one's risk for heart disease (Eckel et al. 2014), though complete removal of these food sources from the diet is not necessary and recent research has brought into question if saturated fat is as "bad" as once believed. Specific types of saturated fats, such as medium-chain triglycerides (MCTs), which get metabolized differently in the body, may actually offer specific health properties. This has given rise to the increased popularity of coconut and coconut products, of which half the fat content comes from MCTs. At the time there is insufficient evidence to support replacing other fats in the diet with MCT-containing foods, like coconut oil. However, these products continue to gain popularity and, to date, no adverse cardiovascular effects have been reported (Bueno et al. 2015).

Unsaturated fats, including mono- and polyunsaturated fats, are considered more "healthful" because of their association with reduced risk for heart disease. Polyunsaturated fats also include sources of the essential fatty acids, omega-3 and omega-6, that are required for certain metabolic functions. Unsaturated fatty acids should make up the bulk of calories coming from fat.

Practical ways to include unsaturated fatty acids include: using olive oil in cooking and salad dressings, placing avocado on sandwiches and salads, adding nuts to oatmeal, eating nuts as a snacks, and regularly consuming fish. Additionally, essential fats such as omega-3 fatty acids are required for the body's anti-inflammatory system to function adequately and help the body to appropriately handle inflammation in the body. See "Practical Implications" for a closer look at Omega 3 fatty acids and athletic performance.

Overall, an athlete should not consume a low-fat diet but rather a diet that is "moderate" in fat (about 20 to 35 percent of total kcal intake) and limit their intake of trans fat, and include sources of mono- and polyunsaturated dietary fat with each meal. Remember, fat not only serves as an energy source during exercise, but also has important roles in maintaining overall health and performance.

Fat Recommendations

Fat can be maligned and some of that simply stems from its name. Yet, fat serves many functions in the body including those essential for performance. Athletes need to be educated on the need for fat in their diet.

Daily Intake

Fat recommendations typically are less precise than those of carbohydrate and protein. While absolute carbohydrate and protein recommendations have been established (expressed as g/kg), an absolute recommended fat intake has not been standardized, though some sports nutritionists aim to ensure an intake of at least 1 g/kg of body weight. Usually, however, fat recommendations are expressed in relative terms (as a percentage) and are calculated after protein and carbohydrate recommendations have been established. This amount ideally should fall within the AMDR for fat based upon the RDA of 20 to 35 percent of calories from fat. Typically, this approach will ensure sufficient intake of fat. This estimation will be illustrated in Chapter 7 on meal planning for athletes.

When an athlete's intake of fat is inadequate, including an insufficient intake of essential fatty acids, there are several risks. First, fat is an important energy source, and endurance and ultra-endurance athletes especially need to be mindful that dietary fat helps restore intramuscular triglycerides that can become depleted during endurance exercise. Inadequate fat consumption may also result in negative health effects, including lowered sex hormone production, and unfavorable blood lipid profiles potentially increasing one's risk for heart disease. Finally, there is a risk of inadequate intake or malabsorption of fat-soluble vitamins with insufficient dietary fat, as well as a risk of deficiency of essential fatty acids.

Fat intakes greater than 35 percent of total caloric intake have potential negative effects as well. First, fat is a very dense nutrient. For an athlete to meet their carbohydrate and protein needs recommended for optimal training and performance, and maintain a high dietary fat intake, they risk an excessive caloric intake that may result in weight gain. If an athlete consumes a high amount of dietary fat while reducing protein or carbohydrate or both to balance calories, then they risk the negative effects of inadequate carbohydrate or protein or both for performance and training. Dietary manipulation of fat that results in a high fat intake has been shown to increase fat oxidation, though this has not been shown to improve athletic performance.

Thus, an athlete should be advised to maintain a fat intake approximating 20 to 35 percent of their calories coming from dietary fat. Too much or too little may result in adverse outcomes. Athletes should be educated on the different types of fatty acids. An emphasis should be placed on incorporating healthy mono- and polyunsaturated fatty acids, to decrease the intake of saturated fatty acids, and limit their intake of trans fatty acids.

Timing of Fat Intake

Again we see that recommendations for the timing of fat intake are affected by the timing recommendations for carbohydrate and protein. Athletes want to avoid high fat intake just before sport. Fat slows the rate of gastric emptying and could impede the delivery of other nutrients to working muscle cells, including that of glucose. Consuming a lot of fat just before exercise may also result in GI distress for some athletes. Thus, athletes are recommended to focus on low-fat food choices before exercise.

Fat consumption should be limited during exercise, especially during high-intensity sports, as well as in efforts to avoid nutrients that delay gastric emptying and impede delivery of carbohydrate to muscles. Some athletes can tolerate small amounts of fat during low- to moderate-intensity exercise, such as with endurance and ultraendurance events, though this has to be established on an individual basis. These athletes should ensure that any fat consumed during exercise is not displacing the more essential carbohydrates, and in some instances protein. Immediately after exercise, athletes want to ensure sufficient intake of carbohydrate and protein, and small to moderate amounts of fat can be appropriate.

Hydration

Function of Fluids

One element of a sports nutrition plan that often goes underappreciated is the importance of proper hydration practices. Athletes may focus on the micro- and macronutrients they should be consuming, but they sometimes neglect their fluid needs. This is an important point of education when working with athletes. Athletes should have a basic understanding of the various functions of fluids in the body, especially as they pertain to exercise. Body water such as synovial fluids allows movement of joints and protects them from damage. Water is what allows transport of nutrients, metabolites, and other substances throughout the body, nourishing cells and excreting waste material.

Perhaps most relevant to athletes, however, is the function of body water in regulating temperature. Working muscles produce metabolic heat that is transferred to the blood and starts to raise the core temperature of the body. In fact, up to 15 to 20 times the amount of heat can be produced during high-intensity exercise in the heat than during rest (Stachenfeld 2014). If the body's core temperature were to rise unchecked, there would be undue cardiovascular strain as well as heat illness, and ultimately death. The body senses increases and decreases in core temperature through a sensor in the hypothalamus that engages thermoregulatory adjustments. When core body temperature increases, there is an increase in blood flow to the skin to dissipate heat via the sweat glands (sweating). The action of sweating is essential to maintain a normal core body temperature, but it effectively reduces the amount of water in the plasma. Dissipating excess heat is extremely important, and sweating is a primary mechanism (along with conduction, convection, and radiation) for heat removal; however, if body water lost via sweat production is not replaced, dehydration and heat injury are likely.

There are many factors that determine sweat rate such as sport type, exercise duration, and intensity. There are environmental determinants of one's sweat rate that include the temperature, humidity, and air motion, and sky and ground radiation. Clothing and equipment that is worn affects an individual's sweat rate. There are other individual characteristics influencing one's sweat rate including body weight, genetic predisposition, heat acclimatization states, and metabolic efficiency (American College of Sports Medicine [ACSM] et al. 2007). While sweating typically accounts for the most significant loss of body water during exercise, there are also respiratory, GI, and renal fluid losses, though these are typically minimal. Recommendations for fluid replacement are outlined later in this chapter.

Assessing Hydration Status

Our bodies are composed of 45 to 75 percent water, with variability due to fat and fat-free mass (fat mass is ~10 percent water, while fat-free mass is ~70 to 80 percent water), age, sex, and race (ACSM et al. 2007). Because of these differences, as well as inter- and intraindividual differences in sweat rate and other rates of water loss, there isn't a single recommended amount of fluids that should be ingested in order to maintain **euhydration**.

Measuring hydration status is best achieved by measuring body water fluctuations. There are precise assessments of hydration status that can be measured in the laboratory involving blood sample collections, but these are not practical for athletes in practice or competition settings. However, established field-tests and collection methods can be done in the athlete's environment.

Simple biomarkers that athletes can use to assess hydration status include urine color and body weight, and while these markers have limitations when used independently, they have greater validity when used in conjunction with each other (Stachenfeld 2014). Athletes should be encouraged to routinely examine the color of their urine in the morning, and they can be provided a urine color chart with which to compare their observation. Athletes can also take their weight first thing in the morning, without clothes on and after having voided, as daily weight will change less than one percent unless affected by hydration status. Tracking several first morning weights (nude, after voiding) will help establish a baseline euhydration status with which they can compare future measurements (ACSM et al. 2007). While these measurements are not as precise as laboratory testing measurements, when taken together they can help an athlete assess one's hydration status.

Athletes who have access to measuring their urine specific gravity (USG) utilizing specialized testing strips will have another method to assess hydration status. Many university and professional teams will regularly measure USG, especially during hot temperatures. A USG of ≤1.020 indicates euhydration, and values higher than this amount indicate the athlete is starting to become dehydrated and rehydration strategies should be implemented.

Put together, fluids are an essential component of any athlete's sport nutrition plan. Athletes should be educated on the function of fluids in the body, have a basic understanding as to what their daily fluid needs are, and how to assess their hydration status.

Fluid Recommendations

Daily Intake

Establishing universal fluid recommendations is not possible due to the significant interindividual variability in the amount of fluids needed. There are multiple influences that affect fluid needs, including variability in sweat rates, dietary habits, and environmental factors that also influence sweat rates. The DRIs have established total water recommendations—125 oz for men and 91 oz for women—and these can be used as an *estimate* of fluid needs. Because food contributes about 19 percent of our fluid intake, actual consumption of fluids from beverages is recommended to be about 101 oz for men and 74 oz for women (Institute of Medicine (U.S.). Panel on Macronutrients and Institute of Medicine (U.S.). Standing Committee on the Scientific Evaluation of Dietary Reference Intakes 2005), though there is great variability in these amounts. Active adults, for example, regularly engaging in physical activity and living in warm, humid climates may have fluid needs as high as 6 L/day (about 203 oz), though this varies greatly by individual (Kenefick and Cheuvront 2012).

All fluids count toward meeting one's needs. Water, juice, milk, and even caffeinated drinks including sodas and coffee contribute towards the DRI fluid recommendations. Caffeine was once thought to result in dehydration, and while it has been shown that in the short term caffeine may result in mild **diuresis**; in the long term caffeine does not seem to negatively affect hydration status (Tarnopolsky 2010). Caffeine will be discussed in greater detail in Chapter 7.

Controversy Over Fluid Recommendations

Assessing hydration status allows an athlete to tailor one's fluid replacement practices to maximize performance and avoid detrimental health effects resulting from dehydration. It is well established that dehydration resulting in loss of up to 5 to 10 percent total body water will negatively impact performance in a variety of exercise types and intensities (Maughan 2012), so athletes should be educated on fluid replacement to avoid such losses. Yet, controversy exists over the effects of dehydration occurring to a lesser degree. Up until recently, there was general consensus and relevant research indicating that dehydration resulting in a body weight loss of 2 percent or more has deleterious effects on performance. The ACSM wrote a position stand in 2007 supporting this assertion and providing fluid replacement recommendations in accordance with prevention of this 2 percent body weight loss; these recommendations were further supported by a position statement made by the ACSM, Academy of Nutrition and Dietetics, and the Dietitians of Canada (ACSM et al. 2007) (ACSM, American Dietetic Association, and Dietitians of Canada 2000).

Recent research has challenged the belief that performance is hindered at a body weight loss of 2 percent. For example, one study examined ultraendurance runners completing a 161 km ultramarathon and found that half of the runners lost more than 2 percent of their body weight, yet this did not seem to have adverse performance outcomes (Hoffman and Stuempfle 2014); another study examined high-intensity intermittent exercise and noted similar findings (Yamashita et al. 2015). Other studies find that athletes who drink in accordance with thirst ("ad libitum") do not experience negative performance effects even with a body weight loss greater than 2 percent. Yet, there are significant methodological concerns of translating the results of these studies into practical recommendations.

Electrolyte Needs

Electrolytes are minerals in the body that help maintain fluid balance through their electrical charge. Calcium, potassium, phosphorous, chloride, and magnesium are all examples of serum electrolytes. Sodium, however, is especially relevant to athletes because sodium can be lost in considerable amounts in sweat during exercise. This can significantly alter fluid balance in the body. The amount of sodium lost in sweat will vary by individual. The typical American diet contains roughly 3.5 g of sodium, and so overall intake is usually not a concern (Kenefick and Cheuvront 2012). However, individuals exercising in very hot temperatures over long periods of time may benefit from electrolyte replacement during exercise. Electrolyte recommendations are discussed in the following section.

Timing of Intake

Until more research is available to replace the current set of recommendations, the ACSM guidelines for fluid replacement will be provided. It is possible that these guidelines will be revised, but until then these standards will determine recommended intake.

Fluid Recommendations Before Exercise

Individuals should commence exercise euhydrated and ensure that plasma electrolyte levels are normalized. This should be achieved several hours before exercise for appropriate fluid retention; this strategy will also allow urination to return to normal output and prevent athletes from taking unnecessary breaks during exercise. Specifically, athletes should aim for 5 to 7 mL per kg of body weight (mL/kg) at least 4 hours before exercise. If the individual still is not producing urine, or urine is very dark in color, athletes should consume another 3 to 5 mL/kg 2 hours before exercise (ACSM et al. 2007). Again, the focus should be to give oneself plenty of time to reach euhydration and allow urine output to return to normal levels. Consuming small amounts of electrolytes, especially sodium, with fluids or foods prior to exercise can support water retention, balance electrolyte levels, and can help stimulate thirst to encourage drinking behaviors.

Fluid Recommendations During Exercise

Most athletes do not experience significant fluid losses until the threshold of about 1 hour of high intensity exercise, or 60 to 90 minutes of steady state exercise (or more). Fluid replacement during exercise below these time frames typically is not warranted; exceptions are for athletes starting exercise in a dehydrated state or exercising in extremely hot and humid climates, or at high altitude. There may be individual variation in sweat rate and sport type that may also warrant fluid replacement within 60 to 90 minutes. A 140 lb male distance runner, for example, may lose up to 2 L of fluids during a 1 hour run due to high metabolic heat production. This emphasizes the importance of knowing an estimate of one's individual sweat rate (such as using pre- and postexercise weight as a measurement tool) as will be described.

Though not uncontroversial, sufficient research supports decrements in performance with a body weight loss of 2 percent or more (Kenefick and Cheuvront 2012). The goal of consuming fluids during exercise is to prevent such body weight losses, as well as to maintain electrolyte balance so that performance is not impaired. There are multiple variables affecting the amount of fluids lost during exercise, including the duration of exercise, intensity, clothing, environmental conditions, individual sweat rates, training status, and acclimatization. Accordingly, there is no singular fluid replacement strategy.

Ideally, athletes get a sense of their fluid losses by tracking weight loss during exercise over various conditions and exercise types (intensity and duration). One way to achieve this is to have athletes weigh themselves in minimal clothing before and after exercise. Assuming that 1 mL of sweat equates to a 1 g loss of body weight, athletes subtract their post-exercise weight from their pre-exercise weight, correcting for urine losses and fluids consumed. See Table 4.6 for an example. As athletes perform these calculations over a variety of contexts (high-intensity versus moderate-intensity training, hot versus cool climates, indoors versus outdoors, etc.) they can start to get an *estimate* of what their typical sweat rates are in various situations. This becomes a very practical and useful tool that athletes can calculate by themselves. While the goal is not to replace 100 percent of fluids lost, as this can lead to feelings of fullness, sloshing, and even

Table 4.6 Calculating sweat rate during exercise

| 1. Take weight before training or competition (minimal clothing, no shoes)
2. Track all fluids consumed during training (in ounces)
3. Take weight postworkout (same clothing, no shoes)
4. Subtract postworkout weight from preworkout weight and convert to ounces (1 lb = 16 oz)
5. Add ounces that were consumed during training
6. Determine hourly sweat rate: divide total ounces lost by hours of training | *Example: Adam exercises for 2 hours and drinks 24 oz*

• Weight preworkout: 135 lbs
• Training fluids: 24 oz
• Weight postworkout: 132.5 lbs
• Difference: 2.5 lbs
• Difference (ounces): 40 oz
• Add training fluids: 40 oz + 24 oz = 64 oz (8 cups)
• Sweat rate = 64 oz/2 hours = 4 cups per hour |

hyponatremia, a reasonable aim can be to prevent fluid losses of 2 percent or more of pre-exercise body weight.

Keeping in mind that there is no "one size fits all" fluid recommendation, a starting point for fluid replacement for exercise greater than 1 hour is approximately 0.4 to 0.8 liters per hour (L/hr). This may be inadequate for individuals who sweat up to 2 L/hr, but in general will be appropriate for most individuals. Within this range, petite female marathon runners who run at a relatively slow pace may be at the lower end of the recommended range (about 0.4 L/hr), and larger-framed male athletes engaging in interval work may benefit from a higher fluid intake (about 0.8 L/hr). Customization of fluid intake is required, and knowing one's individual sweat rate becomes quite useful. Fluids are optimally absorbed when they are ingested at regular intervals, such as every 10 to 15 minutes, though practical considerations of the sport type determine what is most feasible. Avoiding consumption of very large volumes in a short amount of time will also help to avoid gastric distress.

Electrolyte replacement during exercise depends upon exercise type and duration, as well as environmental factors and acclimatization. Sodium replacement is recommended in hot climates when individuals are exercising for several hours, such as in marathon running and other ultraendurance events lasting more than several hours; it may also benefit individuals who are not heat acclimated. An elite marathon runner finishing in less than 3 hours may not need to worry about sodium replacement, for example, but the recreational runner finishing in 6 hours likely will benefit from sodium replacement. Other athletes, including football players practicing for several hours at a time and who are wearing heavy equipment, may lose considerable amounts of sodium during the workout. For those requiring sodium replacement, about 20 to 30 meq/L is a good starting point (ACSM et al. 2007) and can be fine-tuned as needed on an individual basis. This amount can be consumed from most sports drink and in most cases salt tablets are not needed.

A risk of inadequate sodium intake is hyponatremia, or when plasma sodium drops below 130 mmol/L. See "Practical Implications: Hyponatremia" for additional information.

Fluid Recommendations After Exercise

The goal of fluid intake after exercise is to correct for any fluid or electrolyte deficits and to return to euhydration. It is recommended to consume 1.5 L of fluids for every kg (L/kg) of body weight lost, or almost 0.7 L (700 mL) per pound of body weight lost. One kilogram equates to one liter of fluid loss, and the extra 0.5 L is added account for increased urine production that follows a large fluid consumption (ACSM et al. 2007). As with during exercise, it is best to spread out fluid consumption over the next several hours and to avoid a large bolus consumption in order to maximize fluid retention. If an individual has at least 8 to 12 hours until the next exercise bout, they can be more relaxed with their rehydration approach. Those with less than 8 hours typically need a more aggressive rehydration strategy. One way to achieve this is to consume sodium postexercise to help with water retention and stimulate thirst. If sodium is included in postexercise foods consumed, then sodium does not need to be included in a recovery fluid. For individuals who lost a large amount of fluids such as those recovering from an extended exercise bout, adding a little extra sodium to foods or simply choosing salty foods (such as pretzels or soup) can be advantageous.

Putting It Together

Understanding individual recommendations for amount and timing of carbohydrate, protein, fat, and fluid intake is a first step, but being able to integrate these recommendations into practical and relevant strategies is what results in meaningful application. Let's follow a case study of Natalie, a 19-year-old college-level female basketball player. Natalie is 5 ft 9 in. and weighs 145 lbs (66 kg). Natalie is playing in a home game that starts at 8 p.m. Let's see how these recommendations apply to her.

What Natalie Eats Before the Game

Natalie's pregame meal will focus on carbohydrate with moderate protein and small amounts of fat for flavor. Carbohydrate is the main nutrient of focus before activity. Natalie wants to make sure the "gas tanks" are topped off, and carbohydrates are the primary fuel source. Approximately 1 to 4 g/kg should be consumed 1 to 4 hours before exercise. The team is eating at 5 p.m., 3 hours before the game. This means she will aim for 3 g/CHO/kg of body weight, or about 198 g/CHO. Natalie has practiced with different pregame meals and has found that pasta with marinara works for her. She has 2.5 cups of pasta with 1 cup of marinara that has lean ground turkey in it, 1 small basked sweet potato with salsa on it, 8 oz of apple juice, and one banana. Knowing she wanted to get at least 5 to 7 mL/kg of fluids at least 4 hours before the event (or 330 to 462 mL), Natalie made sure that by 4 p.m. she drank her 500 mL water bottle of water. After dinner and leading up to the event Natalie continues to sip on some Gatorade. Heading into the game, Natalie feels great not just physically, but mentally because she knows she has been able to get all of the nutrients she will need to perform her best.

Natalie's Intake During the Game

Other than small amounts of protein that may consumed during endurance and resistance exercise, carbohydrate is the primary macronutrient of interest to meet Natalie's energy needs. Refer back to Table 4.2 for carbohydrate recommendations during exercise. Given that small to moderate amounts of carbohydrate are recommended during moderate- to high-intensity exercise lasting up to 2 hours, Natalie aims for 30 to 60 g of CHO, which will mostly have an effect on the CNS helping to decrease her perception of fatigue. Muscle glycogen will not likely be a limiting factor since glycogen depletion typically occurs after 2 hours and Natalie will be playing for 90 minutes or less. To meet this need Natalie consumes two sport nutrition gels, equaling 60 g/CHO total at half time and drinks 16 oz of water. Of course, this is the case for athletes who start exercise with a "full tank of gas" as Natalie did. This often is not the case with athletes and so carbohydrate consumption during exercise may have to be increased.

Natalie's Intake After the Game

Postexercise nutrition practices are essential for Natalie to experience optimal recovery from exercise; this is the time when the benefits from her hard work are realized. For this to happen, her body needs the appropriate nutrients in sufficient quantities to recovery properly. Given that Natalie will have more than 12 hours to recover (practice the next day is not until 4 p.m.), she has more flexibility in how she meets her recovery nutrition needs. Optimal strategies for her include small frequent meals and snacks instead of one large meal and this extends to rehydration practices as well.

Protein, carbohydrate, and fluids are the primary nutrients Natalie will focus on after her game. Carbohydrate consumed with protein attenuates protein catabolism and stimulates anabolism; consumption of protein with carbohydrate augments the insulin response aiding in glycogen synthesis. These two nutrients, when consumed together, result in a synergistic effect on recovery. The recommended 1.2 g carbohydrate/kg/hr can be hard to attain and so decreasing her intake to 0.8 g carbohydrate/kg/hr in the presence of protein may be a more realistic strategy. This equates to 53 g carbohydrate/hour + 20 g protein, especially in the first hour. Natalie experiences decreased appetite after her intense games and so, for her, meeting her nutrient needs with fluids is more tolerable. Natalie has 20 oz of low-fat chocolate milk (60 g carbohydrate and 20 g protein); this strategy also addresses postexercise protein requirements. When Natalie gets home, she has a peanut butter and jelly sandwich before she goes to bed (55 g carbohydrate and 10 g protein).

Natalie knows from checking her pre- and postworkout weight and calculating her sweat rate that she loses about 0.8 L of fluids per hour. Given her goal of replenishing her fluids 150 percent, she needs to consume 1.8 L of fluids (1.5 hours × 0.8 L = 1.2 L × 150%). She drank about 0.6 L with her chocolate milk; she drinks another 0.6 L over the next 2 hours before she goes to bed.

This case study illustrates all the nutrient needs that need to be met for a particular athlete before, during, and after her competition. The needs of the athlete will vary according to their sport, the duration of activity, estimated intensity, as well as any other individual factors. It is always important to break down each time period (before, during, and after), and go through the different nutrients needed at each stage. The recommendations then need to be customized to the preferences of the athletes and the logistical considerations of the sport.

Practical Application: Should Athletes Supplement with Omega 3 Fatty Acids?

Omega 3 fatty acids have been shown to have cardio-protective effects that reduce the risk for cardiovascular disease, as well as playing a preventive role in the etiology of breast cancer, colorectal cancer, and diabetes in certain populations (Li 2015). The proposed mechanism of action is through the anti-inflammatory properties of these long-chain fatty acids. This has prompted researchers in the exercise field to see if there is a link between Omega-3 fatty acids, particularly EPA and DHA, and inflammation experienced by athletes, and how this might impact performance. Research on this topic is in its infancy and currently includes mostly animal research; preliminary results do support that Omega 3 fatty acids may attenuate delayed-onset muscle soreness (DOMS) and facilitate the recovery process when there is less time available in between exercise sessions (such as two-a-day workouts); other research indicates that omega 3 may promote favorable adaptions in exercise metabolism, which could subsequently improve exercise performance (Mickleborough 2013).

Currently more research is needed before supplementation protocols can be proposed for athletes. There is inconsistency among research methodology that includes variability in the dosages utilized, exercise types studied, populations used, and biomarkers analyzed, as well as a lack of sufficient human studies. There are also inherent risks to Omega 3 supplementation, including risk of contamination of toxins, potential GI side effects, increased risk of bleeding or higher LDL levels, lowered blood pressure (for those at risk of hypotension), and possibly a fishy taste following consumption.

While an optimal dosage of omega-3 fatty acids has yet to be solidified, current research supports a consumption of 1 to 2 g a day of EPA and DHA at a ratio of 2:1 (EPA:DHA), an amount that has not only been designated safe by the Food and Drug Administration (FDA) but is in fact recommended given the essentiality of these fatty acids. The benefits of taking any supplement should outweigh any risks. Currently there is insufficient evidence to support taking omega-3 supplements, especially since these fatty acids can be obtained from the diet; however, some individuals do believe the benefits outweigh the risks, in which case taking a safe dose is less likely to result in negative effects. Any risk associated with omega-3 fatty acid supplementation comes from possible supplement contamination and not from the omega-3 itself. Conversely, athletes can choose to follow the recommended consumption of fatty fish two to three (3.5 oz) servings of fish weekly as part of an overall, balanced diet. This will ensure not only intake of EPA and DHA, but also protein, vitamins, and minerals. Low-mercury, fatty fish include canned light tuna, Pacific salmon, Pollock, and catfish, and given the health benefits of regularly consuming fish, athletes should be advised on strategies to increase their fish consumption.

Practical Applications: Exercise-Associated Hyponatremia

Many athletes may be unaware of the risks of hyponatremia, and so endurance athletes especially should be educated on this medical condition. Technically, what athletes experience is exercise-associated hyponatremia, defined as symptomatic hyponatremia with plasma sodium levels less than 130 mEq/L. This hyponatremia usually occurs in individuals engaging in endurance events lasting longer than 5 hours. These individuals sweat for long periods of time and are losing sodium in their sweat. If they replace their fluid losses with water without consuming foods or beverages containing sodium, extracellular fluids in the body become low in sodium. This causes a shift of water into the cells, and if happening rapidly or severely enough, this can cause congestion in the lungs, swelling of the brain, altered CNS functioning, and ultimately could result in death.

The best way to avoid hyponatremia is to avoid overdrinking. Individuals should be encouraged not to drink more than the amount that they lose, acknowledging that a mild fluid deficit (less than 2 percent body weight loss) will most likely not result in performance impairments. Additionally, individuals who are "salty sweaters" as evidenced by the white salt rings around their forehead and on their shirt (wearing darker shirts can help to identify this), or if they are exercising for more than 4 to 5 hours, should consider electrolyte replacement, particularly sodium. In general, hyponatremia can be avoided by consuming sports drink instead of plain water during prolonged exercise.

The recommended intake of sodium is approximately 20 to 30 mEg/L, though this may need to be customized according to individual sweat rates and sodium content of sweat. This is the sodium amount found in most sports drinks and sport nutrition products. Typically a salt tablet is not warranted, unless the individual is only consuming water and is not consuming sodium-containing foods. In addition, thiazide diuretics and use of nonsteroidal anti-inflammatory drugs (NSAIDs) can increase one's risk for hyponatremia due to interference with the antidiuretic hormone (ADH) that helps regulate fluid balance. Individuals consuming these medications should pay particular attention to appropriate fluid and electrolyte consumption. While this is a very small segment of the athletic population, it is a condition that could be quite serious and athletes in these sports should precautions to avoid.

Definitions

Glycogenesis—the process of adding glucose molecules to glycogen for storage in the liver or in muscle cells, commonly stimulated by insulin.

Muscle cell hypertrophy—an increase in muscle cell size.

Hyperaminoacidemia—having excess amino acids in the blood.

Gluconeogenesis—the production of glucose from noncarbohydrates carbon sources including pyruvate, lactate, glycerol, and glucogenic amino acids.

Euhydration—normal state of body water content.

Diuresis—increased urine production.

References

Ackland, T.R., T.G. Lohman, J. Sundgot-Borgen, R.J. Maughan, N.L. Meyer, A.D. Stewart, and W. Muller. 2012. "Current Status of Body Composition Assessment in Sport: Review and Position Statement on Behalf of the Ad Hoc Research Working Group on Body Composition Health and Performance, Under the Auspices of the I.O.C. Medical Commission." *Sports Medicine* 42, no. 3, pp. 227–49. doi:10.2165/11597140-000000000-00000

ACSM, American Dietetic Association, and Dietitians of Canada. 2000. "Joint Position Statement: Nutrition and Athletic Performance. American College of Sports Medicine, American Dietetic Association, and Dietitians of Canada." *Medicine and Science in Sports and Exercise* 32, no. 12, pp. 2130–45.

ACSM, M.N. Sawka, L.M. Burke, E.R. Eichner, R.J. Maughan, S.J. Montain, and N.S. Stachenfeld. 2007. "American College of Sports Medicine Position Stand. Exercise and Fluid Replacement." *Medicine and Science in Sports and Exercise* 39, no. 2, pp. 377–90. doi:10.1249/mss.0b013e31802ca597

Beelen, M., L.M. Burke, M.J. Gibala, and L.J.C. van Loon. 2010. "Nutritional Strategies to Promote Postexercise Recovery." *International Journal of Sport Nutrition and Exercise Metabolism* 20, no. 6, pp. 515–32.

Beelen, M., N.M. Cermak, and L.J. van Loon. 2015. "[Performance Enhancement by Carbohydrate Intake During Sport: Effects of Carbohydrates During and After High-Intensity Exercise]." *Nederlands Tijdschrift Voor Geneeskdunde* 159, p. A7465.

Bueno, N.B., I.V. de Melo, T.T. Florencio, and A.L. Sawaya. 2015. "Dietary Medium-Chain Triacylglycerols Versus Long-Chain Triacylglycerols for Body Composition in Adults: Systematic Review and Meta-Analysis of Randomized Controlled Trials." *Journal of American College of Nutrition* 34, no. 2, pp. 175–83. doi:10.1080/07315724.2013.879844

Burke, L.M. 2010. "Fueling Strategies to Optimize Performance: Training High or Training Low?" *Scandinavian Journal of Medicine & Science in Sports* 20, Suppl 2, pp. 48–58. doi:10.1111/j.1600-0838.2010.01185.x

Burke, L.M., J.A. Hawley, S.H. Wong, and A.E. Jeukendrup. 2011. "Carbohydrates for Training and Competition." *Journal of Sports Sciences* 29, Suppl 1, pp. S17–27. doi:10.1080/02640414.2011.585473

Eckel, R.H., J.M. Jakicic, J.D. Ard, J.M. de Jesus, N. Houston Miller, V.S. Hubbard, I.M. Lee, A.H. Lichtenstein, C.M. Loria, B.E. Millen, C.A. Nonas, F.M. Sacks, S.C. Smith Jr., L.P. Svetkey, T.A. Wadden, S.Z. Yanovski, and Guidelines American College of Cardiology/American Heart Association Task Force on Practice. 2014. "2013 AHA/ACC Guideline on Lifestyle Management to Reduce Cardiovascular Risk: A Report of the American College of Cardiology/American Heart Association Task Force on Practice

Guidelines." *Journal of American College of Cardiology* 63, no. 25 Pt B, pp. 2960–84. doi:10.1016/j.jacc.2013.11.003

Hoffman, M.D., and K.J. Stuempfle. 2014. "Hydration Strategies, Weight Change and Performance in a 161 km Ultramarathon." *Research in Sports Medicine* 22, no. 3, pp. 213–25. doi:10.1080/15438627.2014.915838

Institute of Medicine (U.S.). Panel on Macronutrients., and Institute of Medicine (U.S.). Standing Committee on the Scientific Evaluation of Dietary Reference Intakes. 2005. *Dietary Reference Intakes for Energy, Carbohydrate, Fiber, Fat, Fatty Acids, Cholesterol, Protein, and Amino Acids.* Washington, DC: National Academies Press.

Jeukendrup, A. 2014. "A Step Towards Personalized Sports Nutrition: Carbohydrate Intake During Exercise." *Sports Medicine* 44, Suppl 1, pp. S25–33. doi:10.1007/s40279-014-0148-z

Kenefick, R.W., and S.N. Cheuvront. 2012. "Hydration for Recreational Sport and Physical Activity." *Nutrition Reviews* 70, Suppl 2, pp. S137–42. doi:10.1111/j.1753-4887.2012.00523.x

Li, D. 2015. "Omega-3 Polyunsaturated Fatty Acids and Non-Communicable Diseases: Meta-Analysis Based Systematic Review." *Asia Pacific Journal of Clinical Nutrition* 24, no. 1, pp. 10–15. doi:10.6133/apjcn.2015.24.1.21

van Loon, L.J.C. 2014. "Is There a Need for Protein Ingestion During Exercise." *Sports Medicine* 44, no. 1, pp. 105–11. doi:10.1007/s40279-014-0156-z

Maughan, R.J. 2012. "Investigating the Associations Between Hydration and Exercise Performance: Methodology and Limitations." *Nutrition Reviews* 70, Suppl 2, pp. S128–31. doi:10.1111/j.1753-4887.2012.00536.x

Mickleborough, T.D. 2013. "Omega-3 Polyunsaturated Fatty Acids in Physical Performance Optimization." *International Journal of Sport Nutrition and Exercise Metabolism* 23, no. 1, pp. 83–96.

Ormsbee, M.J., C.W. Bach, and D.A. Baur. 2014. "Pre-Exercise Nutrition: The Role of Macronutrients, Modified Starches and Supplements on Metabolism and Endurance Performance." *Nutrients* 6, no. 5, pp. 1782–808. doi:10.3390/nu6051782

Phillips, S.M. 2004. "Protein Requirements and Supplementation in Strength Sports." *Nutrition* 20, no. 7–8, pp. 689–95. doi:10.1016/j.nut.2004.04.009

Phillips, S.M. 2012. "Dietary Protein Requirements and Adaptive Advantages in Athletes." *The British Journal of Nutrition* 108, Suppl 2, pp. S158–67. doi:10.1017/S0007114512002516

Poole, C., C. Wilborn, L. Taylor, and C. Kerksick. 2010. "The Role of Post-Exercise Nutrient Administration on Muscle Protein Synthesis and Glycogen Synthesis." *Journal of Sports Science & Medicine* 9, no. 3, pp. 354–63.

Price, T.B., D.L. Rothman, R. Taylor, M.J. Avison, G.I. Shulman, and R.G. Shulman. 1994. "Human Muscle Glycogen Resynthesis After Exercise: Insulin-Dependent and -Independent Phases." *Journal of Applied Physiology* 76, no. 1, pp. 104–11.

Remer, T., D. Krupp, and L. Shi. 2014. "Dietary Protein's and Dietary Acid Load's Influence on Bone health." *Critical Reviews in Food Science and Nutrition* 54, no. 9, pp. 1140–50. doi:10.1080/10408398.2011.627519

Spaccarotella, K.J., and W.D. Andzel. 2011. "Building a Beverage for Recovery from Endurance Activity: A Review." *Journal of Strength and Conditioning Research* 25, no. 11, pp. 3198–204. doi:10.1519/JSC.0b013e318212e52f

Stachenfeld, N.S. 2014. "The Interrelationship of Research in the Laboratory and the Field to Assess Hydration Status and Determine Mechanisms Involved in Water Regulation During Physical Activity." *Sports Medicine* 44, Suppl 1, pp. S97–104. doi:10.1007/s40279-014-0155-0

Tarnopolsky, M. 2004. "Protein Requirements for Endurance Athletes." *Nutrition* 20, no. 7–8, pp. 662–68. doi:10.1016/j.nut.2004.04.008

Tarnopolsky, M.A. 2010. "Caffeine and Creatine Use in Sport." *Annals of Nutrition and Metabolism* 57, Suppl 2, pp. 1–8. doi:10.1159/000322696

Tipton, K.D., B.B. Rasmussen, S.L. Miller, S.E. Wolf, S.K. Owens-Stovall, B.E. Petrini, and R.R. Wolfe. 2001. "Timing of Amino Acid-Carbohydrate Ingestion Alters Anabolic Response of Muscle to Resistance Exercise." *American Journal of Physiology Endocrinology and Metabolism* 281, no. 2, pp. E197–206.

Tipton, K.D., and C.P. Sharp. 2005. "The Response of Intracellular Signaling and Muscle-Protein Metabolism to Nutrition and Exercise." *European Journal of Sport Science* 5, no. 3, pp. 107–21. doi:10.1080/17461390500233607

Wilson, P.B., G.S. Rhodes, and S.J. Ingraham. 2015. "Saccharide Composition of Carbohydrates Consumed During an Ultra-Endurance Triathlon." *Journal of the American College of Nutrition* 34, no. 6, pp. 497–506. doi:10.1080/07 315724.2014.996830

Yamashita, N., R. Ito, M. Nakano, and T. Matsumoto. 2015. "Two Percent Hypohydration Does Not Impair Self-Selected High-Intensity Intermittent Exercise Performance." *Journal of Strength and Conditioning Research* 29, no. 1, pp. 116–25. doi:10.1519/JSC.0000000000000594

CHAPTER 5

Athlete Assessment

The initial encounter(s) with an athlete sets the stage for all future work achieved together. Athlete assessment is a crucial first step in providing appropriate and effective nutrition strategies. The goal of the initial visit is to establish the baseline of the athlete's current position and what the individual's nutrition and performance goals are. The information that is gathered here will dictate the direction of future nutrition guidance.

All individuals looking to improve health and performance through dietary practices should undergo a thorough professional nutrition assessment and provide the practitioner with a detailed understanding of the physical demands of training and competition. This includes an assessment of the periodized training program. Relevant biochemical and medical information is collected by the practitioner, which includes any potential risks or red flags that have nutrition implications. The sports nutrition practitioner then completes an anthropometric assessment and in many cases collects body composition measurements. The sports dietitian will then usually ask about normal daily dietary patterns and intake by using a 24-hour recall or a food frequency questionnaire (FFQ). The individual may also be asked to keep a 3-day diet record prior to the initial consult. Once all of this information is compiled, the practitioner can then formulate pertinent nutrition recommendations to support the goals of the athlete.

Importance of the Athlete Assessment

The link between nutrition and performance has long been established. There is no doubt that optimal nutrition strategies allow athletes to maximize their training efforts and to reach their athletic goals. However, there is no one-size-fits-all approach for nutrition prescription; rather, nutrition recommendations must be individualized. A thorough and comprehensive nutrition assessment will facilitate a customized plan. While this nutrition plan will constantly be revised as the needs of the athlete change (due to training periodization, competition goals, body composition changes and goals, etc.), the nutrition assessment provides a solid foundation for plan development.

Ideally, sports dietitians and nutrition professionals are not working in isolation but rather are part of an athlete's "team" of experts, including but not limited to coaching staff, medical staff, exercise physiology experts, and sports psychologists. When working together, the team can provide cohesive and integrated recommendations. It can be challenging and even counter-productive when athletes are receiving conflicting messages from different providers. Feedback from other team members can be integrated into the nutrition assessment to provide a more comprehensive understanding of the athlete.

The nutrition assessment identifies athletes at risk of nutrition-related problems. Lack of energy for training, impaired recovery, inability to achieve body composition goals, among other challenges faced by athletes can be at least partially the result of poor nutrition practices. The nutrition assessment helps to identify any problematic nutrition habits and can improve many aspects of training and performance. Additionally, information gathered during the assessment will guide interventions and target education as it is relevant to the athlete.

There are many factors affecting a nutrition plan, including but not limited to the sport type of the athlete, the athlete's specialty or sport position, where the individual is in the periodized training schemata, and the training schedule. Individual characteristics of the athlete need to be considered, including age, sex, weight, height, body composition, genetics or physiological information, and health status. Of course, the athlete's nutrition and performance goals must be identified so that nutritional goals can be prioritized.

This is a complex process requiring the collection of many different inputs. This chapter will highlight relevant information that should be gathered during the nutrition assessment as well as identify practical recommendations when it comes times to formulating a plan.

General Health Screening

At the initial consultation, the nutrition practitioner may inquire about a general health screening when working with individuals initiating an exercise regimen; however, this depends upon the individual's overall health and medical history. This component is typically completed by a primary care physician. The sports nutrition expert does not personally clear an individual for exercise, though they should ensure anyone initiating an exercise program has received clearance. If this is not the case, the nutrition professional can refer them to appropriate medical professionals.

Health screenings include a medical history and physical examination. Most individuals can benefit from increased physical activity, but participation should not increase risk of injury or disease. Health screenings can identify individuals who are at increased risk for disease due to predisposing factors, those who are already experiencing a disease state, or those with other special needs and contraindications.

If an individual is found to have a medical concern, this may not necessarily prohibit them from engaging in exercise, but rather may warrant their activity to be medically supervised, or at least modified. At the very least, individuals should complete the Physical Activity Readiness Questionnaire (PAR-Q) as recommended by the American College of Sports Medicine (ACSM). If there is a positive response on the PAR-Q, individuals should be referred to their medical provider. This practice ensures that potential risks are identified and handled appropriately, supporting safe participation in exercise and activity.

Health screenings are relevant to the practitioner who is working with an individual who is starting an exercise regimen or is returning to exercise after taking considerable time off. In these instances, practitioners should know appropriate resources and recommend medical clearance.

Nutrition Assessment of the Athlete

While there are many elements that can be included in nutrition assessments of athletes, there are five components that should be considered foundational, including periodization schemata, biochemical data, medical history, anthropometric information, and dietary assessment. The more information that can be gathered, the more accurate the overall assessment becomes. Before these five elements are considered, some initial information should be collected that can direct further assessments. This includes:

- Sport type: team sport, endurance, strength. Included here is if there are weight requirements or other body weight and aesthetic components.
- Sport position (such as linebacker versus defensive end) or other specialty position.
- Training and competition schedule, including training volume and daily, weekly, and monthly schedules. This will be discussed in this chapter.
- Level of sport: high school, college, professional, and so on.
- Current goals of the athlete, including but not limited to body composition goals and weight management goals, fitness goals, competition goals, improved energy goals, goals for recovery, and so on.

Understanding this information will guide the five main elements of the nutrition assessment and put them into context for the athlete.

Assessment of Training Periodization Schemata

A thorough athlete assessment includes an understanding of the training and competition demands of the athlete. An athlete who works out three to four times a week for 45 to 60 minutes at a time has very different energy and nutrient needs than an athlete training several hours a day, 6 days a week. Many athletes have a training program that includes periodization; that is, a systematic training plan with the aim for the athlete to peak at the most important competition or period of the year. In general terms, this is a way to plan training within the different cycles of competition: preseason, in season, and postseason, and establish appropriate goals. Adjusting the training load, intensity, and volume according to the period of training supports continued adaptations of the body to make gains in sport, while also supporting adequate recovery and preventing plateaus or burnout in athletes. Many athletes break their training down into macrocycles, mesocycles, and microcycles.

The macrocycle of a training program is the year-long plan for the athlete with the goal of achieving peak performance at the most important competition(s). The macrocycle can be divided into distinct mesocycles: the preparatory phase, the competition season (or maintenance phase), and the postseason (or transition phase). Because the preparatory phase can be as long as 8 months for some athletes, it can be broken into an off-season and a preseason mesocycle. Each mesocycle will represent a change in training volume and intensity and may last 2 to 3 months, depending upon the sport and the athlete. The primary principle of periodization is that as the athlete progresses from the off-season into competition season, intensity increases and is then maintained while training volume decreases.

In the off-season, athletes are typically increasing their mileage; this is also where they may address body composition goals. Trying to alter body composition in the preseason or competition season when the athlete is training intensely may result in the nutrition needs not being met and increasing the risk for injury or illness. This will be discussed in greater detail in Chapter 8. Preseason (and for some team sports, the off-season as well) is where the largest volume of training takes place. Other goals of this mesocycle include increasing muscle mass and improving technical skills. Once the athlete is in competition season, training volume decreases while intensity is maintained. This allows fitness to be preserved and avoids excessive fatigue; there is also a focus on the finetuning of skills at this stage. In the postseason, athletes may take some time-off as they recover from the competition season, or choose to cross-train to avoid burnout (mental fatigue).

A microcycle includes the day-to-day training structure and is planned according to where the athlete is in the macro- and mesocycles. The microcycle is where the training components (intensity, frequency, duration) are detailed throughout the week. Knowing these aspects of training is important to understand variations in daily needs.

It is important to know where an athlete is within the training macrocycle in order to provide appropriate nutrition recommendations.

For example, if an athlete is in-season, it may not be in their best interest to address significant body composition goals. The off-season can provide a great opportunity to increase the athlete's sports nutrition education or baseline knowledge so they can apply this knowledge in the preparation and competition season. Thus, knowing where the athlete is in terms of the macrocycle helps tailor effective intervention strategies.

Not all athletes include periodization in their training, though the majority of higher-level athletes do have some form of systematic approach to maximize their training efforts. Wherever an athlete is in the spectrum of training approaches, the sports nutrition professional should be aware of what is the training program and what demands this places on the athlete. Details of the exercise frequency, duration, and intensity should be collected to provide the most appropriate nutrition recommendations.

Biochemical Assessment

Biochemical assessment includes information gathered from blood and urine tests. These data points can provide objective measurements and can support findings from dietary intake. However, the practitioner should keep in mind that while low blood levels may represent low dietary intake, many factors impact biochemical measures, and so there should not be undue emphasis on this information. Disturbances in nutrient absorption and metabolism, diurnal variations, and hydration status can all affect biochemical data that would not be reflective of dietary intake (Fallon 2008). Serum levels of particular nutrients are so tightly controlled through homeostatic mechanisms by the body (such as serum calcium) that blood values may not reflect if dietary intake of a particular nutrient is adequate or not. Additionally, there is a lack of research regarding appropriate blood and urine nutrient values and standards for athletic populations, and in some cases nonactive populations. Therefore, this feedback should only be considered to be one piece of the puzzle.

Due to the cost and invasiveness of biochemical measures, it is not recommended that healthy athletes undergo routine biochemical testing. Routine biochemical testing for iron status in female athletes may be the exception, as well as in athletes who move to or train at altitude since this can impact their iron status, and other high-risk groups (DellaValle 2013); this will be discussed more in Chapter 8.

Medical History

Understanding an athlete's medical history provides insight into any physiological or medical conditions that may impact nutritional intake and nutrient status. This includes assessing for chronic conditions, acute medical concerns, current or past history of nutrient deficiencies, or any other disturbances of digestion and metabolism. Medications an athlete is taking can be relevant especially if there are nutrient–drug interactions or side effects or both of the medications. Finally, getting an understanding of any psychosocial issues (such as depression or anxiety, or other major stressors) an athlete faces, if they are comfortable disclosing, can provide additional perspective into their lifestyle and training regimen.

Anthropometric Assessment

Anthropometrics is the collection of body measurements to gauge growth and development in children and adolescents, as well as appraise body composition in adults. When working with athletes, this includes collecting information on height, weight, skinfold measurements, or other forms of measuring fat mass and fat-free mass. Such measurements not only help assess health status (such as being overweight or underweight), but for athletes with body composition goals, including losing weight or increasing muscle mass, it is essential to have baseline data before changes are recommended. Body mass index (BMI), a ratio of height to weight [ht(m)/wt(kg^2)], is often calculated in clinical nutrition settings as a way to estimate body composition in adults to categorize weight status (underweight, healthy weight, overweight, or obese). BMI does not accurately capture body composition in athletes given their higher muscle mass, which can result in higher BMI values and inaccurate interpretations; thus, BMI has limited applicability in athletes.

When assessing body weight, measurements should be taken at the same time of day, ideally upon waking and after voiding, before any food or beverages have been consumed. Scales should be calibrated regularly according to the manufacturer guidelines or anytime they have been moved. Morning height should be measured using a stadiometer and should be performed by the practitioner, as athletes' self-reported heights can often be inaccurate.

Body Composition

Many athletes have goals to increase muscle mass, decrease fat mass, or both. Often the term "lean body mass" is used when athletes express interest in gaining muscle. While muscle mass and lean body mass are used interchangeably, lean body mass does not only include muscle mass, but also bones, ligaments, tendons, and internal organs. In fact, there is even a small amount of essential fat in the marrow of bones and internal organs that gets included in lean body mass.

There are many reasons athletes seek body composition changes, and appropriate nutrition recommendations for body composition changes are addressed in Chapter 8. Collecting information on body composition as part of the assessment allows for appropriate goal setting and consequent nutrition recommendations. The focus for athletes is typically increasing their muscle mass and decreasing fat mass, and assessing body composition can determine if an athlete's goal for change is realistic. For example, if an athlete already has very low body fat and their goal is to compete in a weight class that is 15 pounds lower than their current weight, it is likely they would have to lose some amount of fat-free mass (muscle) in order to achieve this goal. This may not be desirable. Also, monitoring this information over time (reassessing body composition using the same methodology) allows athletes and practitioners to see if changes are being made and can determine if interventions targeting body composition alterations are successful.

There are various methods for assessing body composition, and practitioners should be aware of the advantages and disadvantages of each. The only way to directly assess body composition is through dissection of the cadaver. Obviously this is not a desirable approach! All other methods are indirect and therefore have certain limitations. Understanding the principles and assumptions underlying the various methods is crucial for accurate interpretation and application. Determining body composition requires identification of different body compartments. Basic, two-compartment models measure fat mass and fat-free mass. Models analyzing additional components such as three-compartment models (measuring fat, bone, and lean mass), or even four-compartment models (measuring bone, adipose, muscle, and other tissues) increase the accuracy of the results. Yet, increasing the number of components measured can greatly increase the cost and reliance upon advanced technology and equipment.

Some assessment tools are more precise than others, and practitioners have to consider variables including what is accessible to them and the athlete, time commitment, cost, availability of published normative data, and training of technician, among other considerations. Keep in mind that all forms of assessment have a margin of error, and this error range needs to be included in interpretation of results.

Skinfold measurements. Collecting skinfold measurements can be a quick and inexpensive way to assess body composition. This method requires a skilled trainer and calibrated skinfold tools, and when these criteria are met, a skinfold assessment on an athlete can be fairly reliable. The practitioner uses calipers to measure folds of skin on specified areas of the body and these values can estimate fat mass and fat-free mass. The skinfold values can be entered into an equation that calculates a percentage of body fat. Since each equation has only been validated on specific reference populations, there is limited applicability to all athletes. There are several types of calipers and procedures that are used in the field, but the protocol developed by "The International Society of Advancement of Kinanthropometry" (ISAK) is considered the gold standard. This method requires implementation by a certified practitioner following a standardized procedure that ensures accurate measurements and minimizes error. Because even a 1 cm deviation in a site measurement can produce significantly different results, using standardized techniques with precise definitions of measurement sites is essential (Ackland et al. 2012). Additionally, when using a prediction equation, the same calipers and technique should be used each time measurements are taken to ensure reliability.

Of note is that ultrasound technology can also be used to measure skinfold. This technique is becoming more common since it decreases trainer error and thus is considered more accurate. However, access to ultrasound technology to be used in this capacity may be limiting, as well as the cost of the technology, depending upon the resources that are available to the athlete.

It is recommended that the sum of the skinfold measurements be determined and used when interpreting results with athletes. A sum of seven or eight measurements is a common calculation. This sum can be compared to normative data that have been established for specific sports. The standard estimate of error for the sum of the skinfold measurements is estimated at about 3 percent when completed using standardized protocols; yet this error is increased to 5 percent when the skinfold measurements are entered into equations to yield percentages (of body fat) due to the inherent error equations introduced into the process. While many athletes really want to know their percent body fat, this can lead to a fixation on the percent number and may result in unhealthy behaviors. Rather, using the sum of the values of the skinfolds can gauge changes and provide useful feedback and does not seem to have some of the qualitative labels (such as "good" or "bad") often seen when using percent body fat.

Overall, skinfold assessments are one of the most frequently used body composition assessment tools in the field. They have the potential to be reliable when performed correctly, though there is still a margin of error that should be included in interpretation of the data.

Bioelectrical Impedance Analysis (BIA). BIA is another practical tool used in the field for assessing body composition. This is a machine that measures electrical impedance, or opposition to the flow of an electric current through body tissues by placement of electrodes on the hands and feet. BIA measures body composition via assessment of total body water, since muscle has a much higher water content compared to fat and water is a conductor of electricity. While fat is an insulator of electricity, the speed at which the electric current passes from one electrode, through the body, and to the other electrode can be used to estimate water content, thus fat-free mass, of the body. BIA has a wider margin of error than other methods, about 3 to 5 percent when conducted under recommended conditions. While the results are not extremely accurate, they can be reliable for the same individual and can assess changes in body composition over time. Accuracy and reliability of BIA requires individuals to be euhydrated because overhydration and dehydration can change total body water estimations. Dehydration may result in a significant overestimation of body fat and overhydration may underestimate body fat. Additionally, athletes should not have recently consumed a large meal or have exercised before BIA assessment because this too can change total body water; therefore, BIA should probably be completed first thing in the morning, after voiding and prior to training or breakfast or both. Strengths of BIA are that it is noninvasive and portable, it can be completed relatively quickly, and does not require a trained administrator. The machine is relatively inexpensive compared to densitometry equipment, though BIA increases in accuracy with added electrodes (4 or even 8 electrodes on hands and feet), which raises the cost of the machine.

Densitometry. Underwater weighing and air displacement plethysmography (ADP) are both assessments of body density. Underwater weighing (UWW), also known as hydrostatic testing, is based upon Archimedes principle that the force on an object submerged equals the weight of the fluid that is displaced. Because lean tissue (bone and muscle) is denser than water, and fat mass is less dense than water, percent fat is calculated based upon the underwater weight of an individual. Residual volume, which is the volume of air remaining in the lungs after a maximal expiration, must be corrected for because air increases buoyancy of the body and failing to account for this leads to overestimation of fat mass. Underwater weighing can be uncomfortable for some individuals and the equipment (especially the tank) is fairly expensive, so this method is not always preferred or accessible. Since the UWW method uses equations to calculate fat and fat-free mass that are based on assumptions regarding the density of bone and muscle tissue, body fat results may be underestimated for many strength-trained athletes and overestimated for individuals with osteopenia or osteoporosis (Ackland et al. 2012).

ADP has recently replaced UWW as a more accessible form of densitometry. ADP, commonly referred to by name given by the manufacturer "Bod Pod," since this is the only commercially available machine measuring ADP, is based upon the same principles as UWW but measures air displacement rather than water displacement. Individuals wear a swimsuit and cap (because clothing and hair displace air thereby reducing one's estimated percentage of body fat) and sit in a small chamber for a few minutes. Body volume and weight are measured, which allows for calculation of body density; this is then entered into an equation to estimate body fat percentage. The Bod Pod has the advantage of being relatively quick, less invasive than UWW (though individuals prone to claustrophobia may find this procedure very difficult), and is relatively accurate with an error range of 2 to 3 percent, about the same as UWW. Because the machine is quite expensive (~$30,000 to $40,000), not many facilities have a Bod Pod, which can limit the availability of the Bod Pod to some athletes. The equations used to calculate body composition are the same as those used for UWW and therefore have the same limitations as described earlier and are not appropriate for all populations, including certain athletic populations.

Dual Energy X-Ray Absorptiometry. Dual Energy X-Ray Absorptiometry, or DXA, measures bone mineral density and for some time has been used in the diagnoses of osteoporosis. DXA is increasingly being used to assess body composition. Two filtered X-ray beams of different energy levels are passed through the body, which are decreased differentially according to the material it passes through. This information allows assessment of fat mass, fat-free soft tissue, and bone density. DXA has advantages in that it is relatively quick, requires little effort on behalf of the participant, does not require a trained practitioner, and is very precise. Limitations include subjection to small amounts of radiation, cost, and availability (it is usually only found in hospital settings). DXA is not affected by hydration status and can be used any time of day, it is also accurate for all populations regardless of training status or bone density but there is some research to indicate that it may be less accurate when estimating body composition in those who are extremely lean, or excessively small or large (Ackland et al. 2012).

Other body composition assessments. Other less common measurement tools of body composition are available. Medical imaging equipment such as computerized axial tomography, or CT scans, and magnetic resonance imaging, or MRI, can be quite accurate. CT creates high-resolution images of the body and can differentiate four different components of the body (bone, muscle, adipose, and other), thus increasing accuracy. However, CT requires exposure to high levels of radiation, more so than DXA, which limits the frequency of use. MRI also produces detailed images of the same four body compartments as CT, but does not require exposure to radiation. Both systems have considerable limitations: they require use of very expensive computer equipment and technology, thus limiting their accessibility; they can induce feelings of claustrophobia in some individuals. Few body composition studies have been conducted using these tools and there lacks normative data with which to compare results (Ackland et al. 2012).

Hydrometry, or use of body water, ultrasound, and 3D photonic scanning are additional methods to assess body composition. Due to limitations that include expense, lack of standardization of methods, and other inaccuracies in the assumptions underlying the techniques, they are not commonly employed to measure body composition. This is not to say they will not become more frequently utilized as some of the limitations are addressed and minimized.

Overall body composition analysis is a fundamental component of the athlete assessment. Knowing an athlete's body composition is essential to understanding if body composition goals are realistic or potentially dangerous. Ongoing body composition assessment provides feedback as to what is successful and what is not in efforts to alter body composition. Continual assessment also allows athletes to see how alterations in body composition affects performance and better define the optimal value that supports performance and health. There is a myth that the lower an athlete goes (in percent body fat), the better the performance; however, understanding body composition feedback can help illustrate the concept of diminishing returns.

Athletes and practitioners must decide upon which method(s) is most realistic based upon available resources and feasibility of different assessment tools. While body composition information can provide useful feedback, athletes and practitioners need to keep in mind body composition is only one aspect of an athlete's training program.

Assessing Dietary Intake

Collecting medical history, relevant biochemical data, and anthropometric information is important, but the dietary assessment is of utmost importance to a sports nutrition professional. Assessing dietary intake, which is then evaluated for nutrition adequacy or inadequacy, can identify risky nutrition-related behaviors, which can help the practitioner determine appropriate dietary recommendations. The assessment also serves as a baseline for making dietary changes, a starting point so-to-speak, and facilitates the prioritization of nutrition strategies. Knowing each athlete's individual behaviors and preferences also allows customization of recommendations, increasing the likelihood of successful implementation. There are many methods to assess dietary intake and it is important to be familiar with different methods and which ones may be most appropriate given the context. Practitioners also need to know limitations of each assessment method so that results are interpreted appropriately.

Assessment of the adequacy of an athlete's diet can be accomplished by looking at previous dietary intake through use of retrospective measures, or by measuring current intake with prospective measures. Both types of assessment have utility in specific situations and sometimes are completed in conjunction with each other to increase knowledge of an athlete's diet and eating patterns.

Retrospective Data

Diet recall. A diet recall requires the nutrition practitioner to ask the athletes to describe everything they consumed (food and beverage) within a defined period, most commonly a 24-hour period. Using a 24-hour recall form, individuals are asked to be as specific as possible, including what was eaten, beverages consumed, estimated portion sizes, brand names when possible, and, specifically when using this method with athletes, information regarding the timing of intake in relation to exercise. Advantages of a diet recall are that it is easy and quick to administer, requires minimal burden on the athlete, and is inexpensive, and because the behaviors under examination took place in the past, behavior was not impacted by the assessment. A limitation of this method is that it relies upon the memory of the athlete, which can significantly affect accuracy, and "yesterday" may not be representative of typical intake. Additionally, a 24-hour recall requires a trained administrator, who is experienced in asking appropriate questions regarding food intake and helping individuals remember certain details. There is a free, online ASA 24 (automated self-administered 24-hour recall) available, though this is more commonly employed in research settings.

Food Frequency Questionnaire. A FFQ uses preestablished food lists and individuals indicate the frequency and amounts of the foods they consume. These surveys can be used as a screening tool to measure and rank the intake of typical foods in the diet; the FFQ also assesses compliance with dietary interventions. Advantages of the FFQ are that it can be self-administered, is inexpensive, provides quantitative information, and—unlike the 24-hour recall—may provide a better assessment of typical intake. A challenge of the FFQ is that, on the one hand, having a more extensive food list helps make the assessment more accurate through inclusion of more foods; on the other hand, having a long food list thus increases the respondent's burden and can negatively impact compliance. Another limitation is that portion sizes can be difficult to estimate with this assessment, and there is also reliance upon memory, which can skew results. Finally, the FFQ has only been validated among certain populations that do not include athletes, thus there is need for a version validated with athletic populations before it can be recommended for use with this population.

Diet history. A diet history combines the 24-hour recall with the FFQ. This is one of the most commonly utilized methods among sports dietitians because it incorporates the strengths of both methods resulting in a more comprehensive assessment of dietary intake. Day-to-day and seasonal variances are captured, and the dietitian is provided with quantitative as well as qualitative information. The limitations of the other methods also apply. Diet history relies upon memory, which can result in inaccurate information, requires implementation by a trained interviewer, and can be more time consuming than either method employed singularly.

Prospective Data

Diet records. Diet records, also known as food logs or food journals, are the most commonly utilized assessments of the current intake of athletes. Athletes record everything that they eat or drink over a 1- to 7-day period, and the practitioner analyzes the information for energy and nutrient content. The more specific the information is regarding selected foods, portion sizes, brand names of foods, times of consumption, the more accurate this assessment becomes. In clinical research, a weighed method that uses scales and computerized approaches is the gold standard, though this is not always practical in nonresearch settings. A duplicate portion method, where individuals gather duplicate samples of the foods and beverages they consume, which are then chemically analyzed for their nutrient content, can also be fairly accurate but are not employed as field methods due to the cost of analysis. In nutrition counseling settings, individuals are encouraged to use household measures (such as measuring cups) to estimate amounts consumed.

Diet records provide detailed information about eating habits, though it may not be representative of typical intake unless this is completed a few times with several months in between to capture seasonal and other variances in dietary patterns. Knowing that the recorded information will be analyzed may impact the dietary choices of the individual, also decreasing representativeness of daily patterns. Because of greater time and effort required from the individual, it is recommended to limit the duration to 3 to 4 days; beyond that, compliance and accuracy may decrease. This method requires the practitioner to have access to a nutrient analysis program and it can take a long time to analyze results. Diet records also require some degree of literacy and nutrition knowledge on behalf of the athlete. Even with these limitations, diet records remain one of the best ways to assess current intake of athletes. The nutrition professional can educate the athlete on how to accurately record food and beverage intake prior to recording; they can also provide the individual with special forms specifically created to teach athletes on correct recording techniques. These interventions can address some of the limitations of diet records. Ultimately, this tool is a practical method to assess efficacy as well as compliance of dietary interventions.

Summarizing Nutrition Assessment

The nutrition assessment is like a puzzle, the more pieces that are available the more complete is the picture of the athlete and their needs. There are instances where not all elements of the assessment are available, such as biochemical data. Sometimes the desirable form of assessment is not accessible, such as measuring body composition with skinfold measurements versus using a DXA. Practitioners must decide what is appropriate to assess and with what methods given available resources. However, of the information that is gathered, there should be awareness of the limitations of each form of assessment so that there is no undue emphasis placed on individual pieces of information. The most effective dietary recommendations will be derived from a comprehensive assessment of all available information and will evolve according to the needs of the athlete.

Definitions

Periodization—the systematic planning of physical training; this involves dividing up the training program into specific phases that each have their own training goals.

Macrocycle—typically a year-long training program with the aim of the athlete "peaking" at the time of major competition. This may include the preparation phase, which comprises the bulk of the training volume; the competition phase; and the transition phase, or the off-season period.

Mesocycle—a defined training period, anywhere from 2 to 6 weeks, within a macrocycle that has specific training adaptations that fit within the overall training plan. The Mesocycle can be used to time training volume and intensity to allow the athlete to peak at competition.

Microcycle—characterizes the training program within a short period, typically a week, and includes the number of workouts within this time frame. This may include light days and hard days and has the aim of realizing acute adaptations to training goals. The microcycle goals depend upon where the athlete is within the macrocycle.

References

Ackland, T.R., T.G. Lohman, J. Sundgot-Borgen, R.J. Maughan, N.L. Meyer, A.D. Stewart, and W. Muller. 2012. "Current status of Body Composition Assessment in Sport: Review and Position Statement on Behalf of the Ad Hoc Research Working Group on Body Composition Health and Performance, Under the Auspices of the I.O.C. Medical Commission." *Sports Medicine* 42, no. 3, pp. 227–49. doi:10.2165/11597140-000000000-00000

DellaValle, D.M. 2013. "Iron Supplementation for Female Athletes: Effects on Iron Status and Performance Outcomes." *Current Sports Medicine Reports* 12, no. 4, pp. 234–39. doi:10.1249/JSR.0b013e31829a6f6b

Fallon, K.E. 2008. "The Clinical Utility of Screening of Biochemical Parameters in Elite athletes: Analysis of 100 Cases." *British Journal of Sports Medicine* 42, no. 5, pp. 334–37. doi:10.1136/bjsm.2007.041137

CHAPTER 6

Meal Planning for the Athlete

Daily Intake

Characteristics of Daily Intake

The daily intake of athletes should be characterized by concepts of balance, variety, and moderation. Balance is found when all three macronutrients are represented in appropriate proportions. There should be a balance of high-quality carbohydrates, proteins, and fats consumed throughout the day to ensure an adequate intake of each; too much of one may displace the other(s). An example of this includes high protein diets that sometimes result in insufficient carbohydrate consumption. This dietary approach can compromise needed sources of glycogen during exercise.

Consuming a variety of foods from each of the food groups each day can help ensure that nutrient needs are being met. Individuals should select a range of foods within each group of fruits, vegetables, whole grains, protein sources, and dairy or dairy alternatives. For example, if an individual eats a banana, an orange, and baby carrots every breakfast and lunch, and steamed broccoli with dinner each night, they are, at least, consuming fruits and vegetables, but they are not getting a *variety* of fruits and vegetables. This same individual could mix berries into their yogurt, raisins in their oatmeal, and have a mixed fruit smoothie as a snack as a means to incorporate a greater assortment of fruits. They could choose salad as a side dish, include peppers and zucchini when grilling meat, and add tomatoes to wraps and sandwiches to get a greater variety of vegetables. More variety represents a greater diversity of nutrients. One way to present this concept to individuals is to suggest that the more color, the better. Of course, this applies to fruits and vegetables, and not to brightly colored Fruit Loops!

Moderation is a concept pertinent to athletes, though their challenges may be slightly different from those of less active individuals. Moderation means avoiding excess, or extremes, and applies to food and beverage choices. Too much of anything will eventually result in negative effects, and this includes an excessive intake of just about any food or food group. Most common among Americans, which includes athletes, is an excessive intake of solid fats and added sugars, or SoFAS. Solid fats are fats solid at room temperature; in the American diet, this includes grain-based desserts, pizza, cheese, and processed meats. Solid fats are associated with increased risk for certain chronic diseases. Foods with added sugars include sodas, energy drinks, sports drinks, grain-based desserts, and sugar-sweetened fruit drinks. These foods tend to have a high amount of empty calories; that is, calories with little or no nutrient value and also associated with increased risk for chronic disease as well as dental caries. Sports drinks may be appropriate for athletes but are specific to exercise needs; athletes typically do not need sports drinks to "fuel" their television watching.

The 2010 Dietary Guidelines for Americans have recommended reducing the intake of SoFAS, as well as excess sodium consumption, though it appears that the upcoming Dietary Guidelines (that have yet to be available at the time of publication) will have a reduced focus on fat. It is astonishing that 35 percent of the calories in the American diet, equivalent to about 800 calories, come from SoFAS (U.S. Department of Health and Human Services, U.S. Department of Agriculture, and U.S. Dietary Guidelines Advisory Committee 2010). Foods high in SoFAS not only contain nutrients that can be harmful to health, including trans fat and added sugars, but these foods tend to be low in the nutrients that promote overall health, such as vitamins, minerals, and fiber. By reducing intake of SoFAS and increasing the amount of nutrient-dense foods, individuals including athletes can increase the overall **nutrient density** of their diet. This concept of moderation even applies to what are considered "super foods," that is, foods with a high nutrient density, though the risk of consuming too many healthy foods is much less common than overconsumption of less healthy foods. There is such thing as "too much of a good thing." Foods like kale, blueberries, and quinoa are often touted as super foods because they have a high nutrient content in relation to the calories they contain. Even kale, for example, could be problematic in extremely high amounts. Kale is high in vitamin K, and too much vitamin K could interfere with certain medications including blood thinning medications.

While nutrient toxicities from food sources are rare, a more common concern of consuming excessive amounts of certain foods is that a high intake of one food may result in an inadequate intake of another. Individuals who eat too many SoFAS have less room in their diet for more nutrient-dense foods. Balance is key to avoiding excessive intakes of any one nutrient, and to ensure adequate intake of a variety of foods. One can see how the concepts of balance, variety, and moderation are overlapping principles to be applied to daily food intake.

Discretionary Calories

While the concepts of balance and variety can be applied to athletes as they are to their nonactive counterparts, moderation may look differently for athletes than for sedentary individuals. This is in part because athletes generally have higher energy needs due to their higher energy expenditure. For example, a 150-pound sedentary woman may need 1,650 kcal to maintain her weight. A 150-pound elite female mountain biker who trains several hours a day may need more like 2,600 kcal a day, which is a 63 percent increase in calories. The female mountain biker will have a greater need for certain vitamins, minerals, and fiber; additionally, she will need added energy from carbohydrates and will have higher protein needs. These increased needs should be primarily met with nutrient-dense sources of carbohydrates, proteins, and fats. However, even after meeting these increased needs, athletes may find they still have some calories "left over." These can be considered *discretionary calories*, or calories that go toward the total calorie allowance after meeting recommended nutrient intakes, and these calories can be chosen with more flexibility.

For the female mountain biker who meets her increased nutrient needs, she may still have another 175 kcal, for example, which go toward meeting her energy needs. She may choose to "spend" these calories on a cookie, for example. Discretionary calories can be less nutrient dense than the foods comprising the foundation of her diet. Discretionary calories may be appropriate in limited amounts as long as nutrient needs are being met and total caloric intake is not exceeding recommended intake. Athletes may have more room for discretionary calories in their diet than less active individuals, but they should be counseled to choose these calories wisely. The nutrient composition of unhealthful foods can still be detrimental to health if consumed in high amounts. Additionally, discretionary calories needed to fulfill total energy needs can be healthful choices, and certainly do not *need* to come from empty calories. This can be an important point of education when working with athletes, as their perception may be that they are allowed a much higher amount of dietary sugar and saturated fat than is actually recommended.

Discretionary Calories: Alcohol Recommendations for Athletes

Alcohol is one of the most commonly consumed recreational drugs world-wide, and the United States has one of the highest rates of alcohol consumption in the world. While there are sports professionals and sports' governing bodies that advise against alcohol consumption by athletes, this may not be a realistic strategy given the pervasive presence of alcohol in society. Thus, it may be more prudent for the sports nutrition practitioner to give athletes guidance on safe alcohol consumption practices.

The U.S. Dietary Guidelines define a "drink" as 12 oz of beer, 5 oz of wine, or 1.5 oz of an 80-proof hard alcohol and goes on to recommend that, if individuals choose to drink, they should do so in "moderation," which is further defined as one drink a day for women and two drinks a day for men. Binge drinking, however, is defined as the amount of alcohol that results in a blood alcohol concentration of 0.08 g percent or higher. This typically results from the consumption of four drinks in women, or five drinks in men, in 2 hours or less. Binge drinking can also result in high-risk-taking behavior, lower inhibitions, alcohol poisoning, and neurological damage, among many other risks. Alcohol is considered a banned drug according to the National Collegiate Athletic Association (NCAA) in certain sports. All individuals should be counseled on the dangers of high alcohol consumption.

Looking at alcohol consumption among athletes, most research has been conducted in collegiate populations. Results indicate that college athletes drink more than their peers, and they are more likely to binge drink (Ford 2007) and males more so than females. Binge drinking appears to be more common among team sports versus teams made up of individual athletes, such as cross-country running or gymnastics and it is this behavior of excessive alcohol consumption that is of greatest concern.

Regarding the effects of alcohol on performance, there is variability in the research depending upon the amount and type of alcohol consumed, timing of consumption, type of exercise, and individual tolerance for alcohol. In general, alcohol consumption at low-to-moderate doses does not improve performance (as once was thought) but may have a negative effect on endurance performance; there does not seem to be an effect on strength output (Barnes 2014).

The majority of research has examined the effects of alcohol on recovery from exercise, since this most closely mimics the behaviors of athletes. If consumed in large amounts, alcohol can increase diuresis (urine output) and negatively impact hydration status; this does not seem to be the case at lower alcohol intakes. Additionally, high alcohol consumption has been shown to displace more beneficial complex carbohydrates that should be consumed and, as an effect, may impair muscle glycogen resynthesis. That is, high alcohol intake may decrease the intake of dietary sources of carbohydrates that are needed to replenish glycogen stores. Studies that have looked at athletes who consume adequate carbohydrates *and* a large amount of alcohol find that overall energy intake in these situations tends to be quite high and can negatively affect energy balance. Alcohol has 7 kcal/g, thus contributing substantially to total energy intake. Other aspects of the recovery process are negatively impacted by high alcohol intake. There may be negative effects on the immune system as well as hormonal alterations that can result in mood and sleep disturbances. Sleep disturbances alone can be detrimental to performance, especially if high alcohol consumption the night before a competition or event compromises sleep. There is also preliminary research indicating alcohol can impede protein synthesis (Barnes 2014).

Put together, sports nutrition practitioners should work with athletes on educating them on safe and appropriate alcohol consumption. Drinking heavily the night before an event can have negative effects, as can alcohol consumption immediately prior to exercise. Having low-to-moderate alcohol intake following exercise is considered safe, though athletes should ensure an adequate intake of recommended recovery nutrients. Alcohol intakes at higher amounts can impede the recovery process or lead to excess weight gain and athletes should be discouraged from these practices.

MyPlate Illustrates Concepts of Balance, Variety, and Moderation

Very basic tools illustrating the concepts of balance, variety, and moderation are presented through the U.S. Dietary Guidelines and include the MyPlate icon. Available on the United States Department of Agriculture's website www.choosemyplate.org, MyPlate is a great visual for a healthful eating approach. As shown in Figure 6.1, MyPlate graphic breaks the plate into three components with specified proportions. Fruits and vegetables comprise one-half of the plate, and whole grains and lean protein options comprise one-fourth of the plate each (the MyPlate graphic does not specify whole grains and lean proteins, just grains and proteins, but this is a great opportunity to educate individuals on the benefits of making whole grain and lean protein choices).

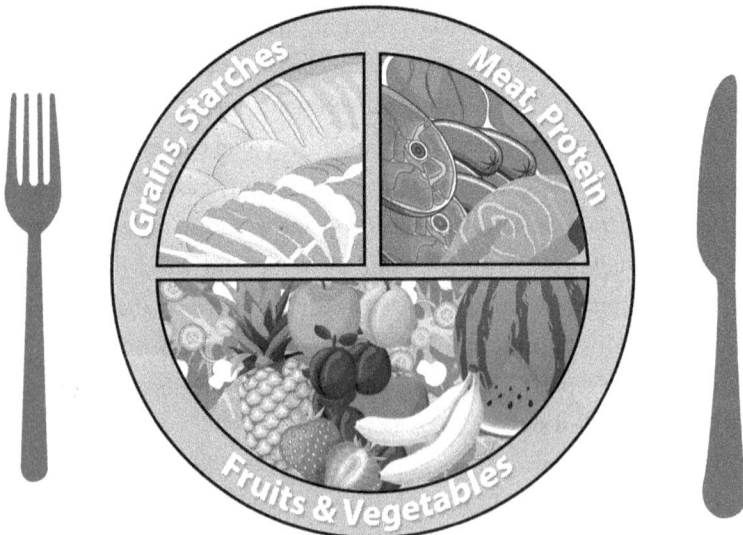

Figure 6.1 The plate method

Athletes can be educated on how to use this template as a way to gauge their own meals. For athletes with low-to-moderate activity, the proportions of MyPlate are appropriate. Athletes with moderate activity levels will better meet their energy needs with proportions of one-third each fruits and vegetables, whole grains, and lean proteins; for athletes with high levels of training a plate comprising half whole grains, one-fourth vegetables, and one-fourth lean proteins is needed in order to meet their increased energy needs. These plate visuals can be a great tool for athletes to assess balance of food groups as well as proportionality of these nutrients wherever they go.

Nutrition Implementation: Translating Numbers to Behaviors

Providing athletes with the fundamentals of sports nutrition and educating them on what their daily intake should be is one thing; it is a completely different skill to be able to assist athletes in implementing the knowledge that has been imparted. Helping athletes make sense of the numbers and how they translate to behaviors is essential for successful adoption of nutrition recommendations.

Chapter 2 demonstrates assessment of energy needs, and Chapter 4 breaks down the specifics of carbohydrate, protein, fat, and fluid recommendations. This information can be compiled into an individualized nutrition plan that provides the recommended macronutrient and fluid amounts specific to the athlete. Athletes can be taught how these nutrients are balanced appropriately, are consumed from a variety of food sources, and to apply the concept of moderation to their food choices. The next step is to teach athletes how to execute these recommendations in a practical and meaningful way.

Supporting athletes in successful implementation of dietary practices can be accomplished in a number of ways. Some sports dietitians have preestablished meal plans at different calorie levels, and these can be tweaked and changed to meet an individual's specific macronutrient needs. Using preestablished meal plans can be a helpful way to simply demonstrate what healthful dietary patterns look like. Some athletes simply have no idea what a "healthy" daily intake looks like, and preset meal plans provide this visual even if the athlete does not follow that specific plan. Some athletes need significant dietary changes, which can be assessed from baseline data such as a food journal or a 24-hour dietary recall or both. Take, for instance, a high school or college athlete who eats a lot of fast food and consumes very few fresh foods. If very few of their existing behaviors are healthful, a preestablished meal plan that is customized to one's likes and dislikes can be a useful approach. Other athletes may be relatively close to meeting their needs or are already engaging in healthy behaviors. In these cases, the athletes' current dietary patterns are analyzed for nutrient and energy content, and can then be adjusted and modified to meet their specific nutrient needs. Other times, a combination of approaches can be used such as creating and strategizing meal ideas for an athlete who skips breakfast.

The closer the practitioner can incorporate the athlete's current daily intake into their suggestions, the more likely the recommendations will be successful. Nutrition plans that resemble typical daily intake face fewer obstacles because there is some familiarity for the athlete. This illustrates the importance of a thorough nutrition assessment and a familiarization with an athlete's usual dietary habits. Dietary preferences, dislikes, allergies or intolerances, and potential religious practices or food ethics are all relevant to developing a nutrition plan that is customized to the individual.

To apply these concepts and translate them into dietary recommendations, let us look at an example. Brian is a 27-year-old Nordic cross-country skier competing at the international level. He weighs 150 lb (69 kg), and is 5 ft 10 in (70 in). Based upon the macronutrient recommendations outlined in Chapter 4, Brian's needs are outlined in Table 6.1.

Brian needs to understand how to translate the number of grams of carbohydrate, protein, and fat to food choices. First, Brian's energy needs are established, and according to the Cunningham equation, Brian needs ~3,700 kcal/day. Based upon Brian's training volume, he needs 8 g carbohydrates/kg/day, equaling 2,184 kcal/day from carbohydrates. His protein needs are 1.4 g/kg/day, resulting in 380 kcal/day from protein. If we estimate that he needs 1 g fat/kg/day (which would be a minimum amount of fat), then he will consume 612 kcal/day from fat. The sports nutritionist can go through Brian's daily intake from the dietary assessment and compare current intake with recommended intake values. Brian

Table 6.1 Dietary recommendations for Brian Nordic Skier

Wt: Ht:	150 lb (68.2 kg) 70 inches

Calories	RMR = 500 + 22(FFM) − Cunningham equation
	    = 500 + (22 × 61.4 kg)
	    = 1,851 kcal
	1,851 kcal × 2.0 (activity coefficient based upon heavy activity; see Table 2.2) = 3,702 (3,700)
	3,700 kcal/day

Carbohydrate	8 g/kg/day = 8 g × 68.2 kg = 546 g of carbohydrate a day = 2,184 kcal from carbohydrate a day
Protein	1.4 g/kg/day = 1.4 g × 68.2 kg = 95 g of protein a day = 380 kcal from protein a day
Fat	1.0 g/kg/day (minimum) = 1.0 g × 68.2 kg = 68 g of fat a day = 612 kcal from fat a day
Calories from recommended carbohydrate, protein, and fat	= 2,184 kcal + 380 kcal + 612 kcal = 3,176 kcal
Discretionary calories	= Total calories minus recommended calories from macronutrients = 3,700 kcal − 3,176 kcal = 524 kcal/day

can then be shown how to modify meals and snacks that might require adjusting in order to align with timing recommendations, such as adding a snack after training but prior to dinner. Along with this recommendation, he can be educated on nutrient-dense food choices for snack ideas.

Brian will then have 524 remaining "discretionary" kcal once he meets his macronutrient needs with nutrient-dense foods. If Brian had a goal of decreasing fat mass, he might choose to cut out some of these discretionary calories, and over a month's time he could feasibly lose about 1–4 lbs of fat mass given appropriate dietary strategies for weight loss (see Chapter 8). If Brian is working toward weight maintenance, some of these calories may be allocated for alcohol consumption, or a treat or dessert that he enjoys. However, it would not be advisable for Brian to "spend" all of these 524 calories on alcohol or treats; this could significantly reduce the nutrient density of his diet and potentially impact his health. Rather, he should be educated on including other nutrient-dense choices. Given that his initial fat intake was estimated at 1 g/kg, this could also be an appropriate nutrient to increase with an emphasis on healthful fat choices. The concept of discretionary calories is important to understand. An athlete first should meet their carbohydrate, protein, and then fat needs with nutrient-dense choices; by calculating these values, athletes can have an idea of what is "left over" for "treats" and less nutritious choices.

Nutrition education is essential for athletes to understand the connection between the foods that they eat and their performance. In fact, many coaches and training staff members believe nutrition knowledge was a significant determinant in an athlete's nutrition intake (Heaney et al. 2008). Yet, imparting knowledge is just one component of nutrition intervention with athletes; athletes need to implement this knowledge in their daily lives in order to receive the benefits of sound nutrition practices.

Barriers and Strategies to Proper Nutrition Practices

Athletes identify many challenges they face when attempting to implement sound nutrition principles. Limited financial resources is a frequently cited reason for improper nutrition habits, since many athletes believe eating healthier costs more money and so they opt for cheaper, lower-quality foods. The practitioner needs to have a general sense of an individual's food budget in order to provide realistic recommendations. Athletes can also be educated on meal planning techniques that can result in significant cost savings, including utilizing weekly sales at their local grocery store, buying in bulk when possible, planning meals out in advance to prevent unnecessary trips to the store, and avoiding excessive eating out. Sports nutrition professionals should have a basic awareness of meal planning tools to help athletes eat healthy in a cost-effective way that works with their budget.

Time is another resource that may limit athletes' abilities to follow healthy eating guidelines. Many athletes are working or are students, or both, on top of their rigorous training schedules. They may not have the hours they think they need to spend in the kitchen each day preparing healthy foods. Consequently, some athletes choose highly processed, packaged foods that may not meet their nutrient needs. This is another misconception of healthy eating that can be addressed. Meal planning can be used in this context as well, since meal planning can save time by prepping some items ahead of time and using batch cooking methods that allow for several meals to be made at once. Athletes can be shown simple meal preparation techniques and short cuts for preparing healthy foods; for example, teaching athletes easy meals they can make with minimal time using frozen vegetables, quick prep whole grains, and lean protein can prevent excessive fast food consumption.

Athletes can also be educated on healthy menu options when eating out. Meal planning and basic kitchen skills can prevent unnecessary fast food stops, but sometimes eating out is unavoidable, such as when traveling for competitions. Other social and lifestyle factors may result in athletes eating out on a regular basis. Many fast food restaurants offer healthy choices that can meet an athlete's nutrient needs. Athletes can be taught how to read menus to discern appropriate choices, as well as how to access online nutrition information from restaurant chains. Providing education on eating out healthfully can be an essential component of working with some athletes.

Many athletes benefit from guidance on how to use nutrition labels and information available on the Internet to educate themselves on selecting nutrient-dense foods. There is a lot of information available to consumers if they know where to find it. Athletes who can use nutrition labels and available nutrition information to compare products and make appropriate choices will have a tool set that they take with them wherever they go.

Other barriers to healthful eating practices experienced by athletes include (lack of) support from other members of the household, social influences, stress, and other emotions. For example, some athletes may cope with stress by "comfort" eating. These challenges can be addressed by a sports nutrition professional and athletes can be referred to appropriate resources if needed, but only if the practitioner is aware of these issues. Basic assessment of emotional health is to be an ongoing part of the discussion with an athlete. When issues are identified and worked through, an athlete is more likely to successfully implement nutrition recommendations.

Competition Diet

The importance of developing a nutrition strategy for competition can often be an underappreciated component of the athlete's diet. Of course, the day-to-day nutrition practices are key to helping an individual train hard and develop as an athlete. But the months, and even years, of commitment to sport and training mean very little to performance goals if nutrition practices impede an athlete from reaching one's athletic potential at competition. A marathon runner who "bonks" at mile 20 because of improper nutrition planning, or a bobsled athlete who loses focus on their second competition run because of poor carbohydrate intake and timing show how crucial dietary strategies are to peak performance. Every athlete looking to compete in their respective field, whether it be the recreational cyclist looking to complete their first century ride for fun, or the elite taekwondo athlete competing in World Championships, should have a nutrition plan for competition.

Ensuring Adequate Nutrient Availability

Preparation for race day should not only take place on the day itself, but can begin up to a week before the event (or sometimes longer) and should be planned out even further in advance. Additionally, training is typically adapted to prevent excessive fatigue such as through a tapering regimen. Nutritional strategies are also essential for preventing fatigue. Glycogen depletion and dehydration are two potential causes of fatigue and are preventable through intentional practices.

Knowing that carbohydrate is a primary fuel source for exercise, athletes want to ensure their "gas tanks" or glycogen stores are full. Starting an event with low glycogen stores can result in early fatigue and can become a limiting factor in performance. For events lasting up to 90 minutes, normal glycogen stores are sufficient, though for events lasting longer, carbohydrate loading may be recommended (see section on "Carbohydrate Loading"). Glycogen stores can be normalized (assuming they were depleted from training) within a 24- to 36-hour period with high carbohydrate intake (7 to 10 g/kg/d) and no additional exercise (Burke et al. 2011). While a section in Chapter 4 "carbohydrate recommendations before sport" recommends 1 to 4 g/kg of body weight in the 1 to 4 hours before the event, even the day preceding the event should be used to ensure adequate glycogen content. These meals should be rich in complex carbohydrates balanced with moderate protein and healthy fats. Meals should be lower-residue foods, which include the avoidance of excess dietary fiber and other substances that may cause gastrointestinal distress such as spicy and high fat meals. Maintaining no to low activity will also support glycogen repletion.

It seems athletes are aware of the importance of carbohydrate-rich meals the night before an event as exemplified in the proverbial "pasta dinner" consumed by many athletes. When educating athletes, it is helpful to discuss all the different sources of carbohydrates, including fruits, starchy vegetables, milk, yogurt, and all types of grains. There is nothing magical about pasta. If athletes prefer pasta than that can be a convenient option, though a high carbohydrate meal can be prepared that focuses on other types of food. Whichever sources of carbohydrates the athlete includes, these foods should be familiar and well tolerated. Table 6.2 provides a sample of a carbohydrate-rich meal consumed the night before the event for a 55-kg female distance runner that provides roughly 4 g/kg.

Hydration practices also have an impact on race day performance. Dehydration results in feelings of fatigue among other risks depending upon the degree of dehydration. Specific hydration strategies before

Table 6.2 Carbohydrate-rich meal the night before an event for a 120-lb/55-kg female distance runner

Food	Carbohydrate (g)	Calories (kcal)
1 1/2 cups steamed butternut squash	32	123
1 1/2 cups couscous	55	264
3 oz grilled chicken	0	98
1 ear corn on the cob	20	80
1 dinner roll	15	87
1 tbsp raspberry preserves	13	53
1 cup pineapple chunks	22	83
10 oz 100% grape juice	48	175
Total	205	963

Note: Tbsp = tablespoon; oz = ounce.

exercise have been discussed (see Chapter 4, fluid recommendations before exercise); specifically, athletes should aim for 5 to 7 mL per kg of body weight (mL/kg) at least 4 hours before exercise. If the individual is still not producing urine, or it is still very dark in color, they should consume another 3 to 5 mL/kg 2 hours before exercise (American College of Sports Medicine et al. 2007). However, to avoid the consumption of excess fluids in the hours before an event that could result in unnecessary restroom breaks during competition, athletes should be euhydrated heading into the day of competition. This can be achieved by monitoring urine output and color (think clean, clear, and copious) so that going to sleep the night before the event they are in good hydration status. This will prevent the need for "catch up" hydration practices on the day of the event.

Carbohydrate Loading

Carbohydrate loading is a performance- enhancement strategy that intentionally increases muscle glycogen stores beyond normal values in order to delay fatigue during a critical performance. Carbohydrate loading was first examined in 1967 by researcher Bjorn Ahlborg who found that physically active, though not specifically well trained, individuals could supercompensate their glycogen stores over a 7-day period (Bergstrom et al. 1967). The protocol in these initial studies included a 3-day glycogen depletion period during which individuals engaged in exhaustive exercise and consumed a low carbohydrate diet. The following 3 days aimed for supercompensation of muscle glycogen by consuming a high carbohydrate diet and engaging in little to no physical activity. Indeed, biopsies reflected increased muscle glycogen content, and endurance performance was improved in these athletes (Bergstrom et al. 1967).

This protocol does not represent a practical nor ideal strategy for athletes. The glycogen depletion phase includes completing exhaustive exercise, which may not be conducive to an athlete's tapering plan. The glycogen depletion phase has other potential negative effects to the athlete, including potential increased risk for illness or injury, and other mental and cognitive effects of being on a low carbohydrate diet that includes irritability and decreased mental acuity (Sedlock 2008).

Fortunately, in the time since these initial studies, it has been shown that athletes can increase their muscle glycogen stores without requiring the glycogen depletion phase of the original carbohydrate-loading procedure. Sherman et al. in 1981 demonstrated an almost doubling of muscle glycogen content by following an exercise tapering program and consuming a high carbohydrate diet (70 percent of calories from carbohydrate) for 3 days in the absence of glycogen depletion. This is a much more "user-friendly" approach (Sherman et al. 1981). While some studies demonstrate greater glycogen storage following glycogen depletion, this process may not be warranted for some athletes due to the resulting fatigue and disruption it can have on the training and taper program.

Supercompensation of glycogen stores appears to benefit athletes competing in events lasting longer than 90 minutes; otherwise, glycogen stores can be normalized within a 24-hour period given reduced training and adequate intake and is sufficient for sports of shorter duration (Burke et al. 2011). It has been shown that 7 to 12 g/kg/d is needed to achieve maximal glycogen storage. There is no singular protocol that results in optimal storage, but rather a variety of strategies are possible. Many studies have utilized a three-day loading period, although other studies have shown that 1 day of high carbohydrate intake (10 to 12 g/kg/d) paired with physical inactivity can result in equally high glycogen storage (Bussau et al. 2002; Fairchild et al. 2002). Additionally, while it was thought that the high carbohydrate intake had to take place in the days immediately prior to competition, updated research has demonstrated that a high carbohydrate intake followed by up to 5 days of moderate carbohydrate intake (50 to 60 percent of total energy intake) maintained supercompensated carbohydrate stores (Arnall et al. 2007; Goforth et al. 2003). Thus, there are various approaches athletes can take to maximize their glycogen content, which can minimize interference with their training program and preparation for competition. Table 6.3 illustrates a sample day of carbohydrate loading for a 70-kg male cyclist providing 8 g/kg/d.

It is interesting that many endurance athletes seem to be aware of the benefit of carbohydrate loading, though only some of these athletes actually implement the recommended protocol. In a study that looked at ultraendurance male cyclists competing in a 210 km race (~134 miles), 57 percent of the athletes reported carbohydrate loading; yet, of these

*Table 6.3 Sample one-day meal plan for a 154 lb/70 kg male cyclist.
Provides 8 g/kg/d*

Food	Carbohydrate (g)	Calories (kcal)
Breakfast	**168**	**757**
2 slices whole wheat toast	48	240
2 tbsp strawberry jam	26	100
1 banana	23	90
6 oz nonfat fruit yogurt	32	162
12 oz orange juice	39	165
Snack 1	**60**	**302**
Chocolate chip Clif Bar	44	240
1 cup grapes	16	62
Lunch	**129**	**665**
1 × 6 in. pita bread	35	170
2 tbsp hummus	5	50
3 oz deli meat	2	77
2 slices tomato	1	8
3 slices romaine lettuce	0	1
1 cup fresh mango slices	25	99
1 oz sourdough pretzels	25	120
8 oz apple juice	36	140
Snack 2	**49**	**260**
1 cup applesauce	48	180
1 string cheese	1	80
Dinner (stir fry)	**152**	**817**
1 1/2 cup rice	80	363
4 oz tofu	3	93
teriyaki sauce	6	32
1 1/3 cup mixed vegetables	24	120
1 baked potato	26	113
2 tbsp salsa	1	10
1 cup nonfat milk	12	86

Snack 3	33	190
1 cup toasted oat cereal	20	100
1 cup milk	12	86
Total	590	2,991

Note: Tbsp = tablespoon; oz = ounce.

individuals, only 23 percent were actually consuming the minimum amount of recommended carbohydrate (7 g/kg/d) for CHO loading (Havemann and Goedecke 2008). This demonstrates that while athletes may be aware of the importance of carbohydrate for endurance events, their knowledge of implementing actual research-based recommendations may be limited. Hence the importance for appropriate nutrition education by a qualified practitioner.

There are potential side effects with carbohydrate loading that include bloating and GI discomfort. Water is stored with glycogen and so water retention is a common experience; this can lead to feelings of fullness and heaviness and this will be especially relevant to weight-bearing athletes, such as runners, compared with athletes that are weight supported, such as cyclists (Sedlock 2008). Athletes should experiment with carbohydrate loading prior to competition to become familiar with their own response to the process. In general, though, many athletes believe the benefits outweigh the costs, especially when steps are taken to minimize any potential discomfort.

Race Day: No Surprises

One of the most important principles for race day is to have no surprises pertaining to nutrition. Athletes should train like they race and race like they train. The day of the big competition is not the time to experiment with a new food, since this could have deleterious results. Even if the race venue is serving delicious-looking pancakes, if that athlete is not accustomed to eating pancakes before racing they may find themselves making unnecessary restroom breaks. Other athletes eat pancakes before the race and achieve their best performance. There is nothing wrong, or right, with pancakes, it is all about what the athlete is used to. There should be no surprises on race day.

Being prepared for competition requires planning well in advance. Athletes should be familiar with the physical demands of the event as much as is recommended according to the training plan. Some athletes will actually complete the competition event in their training, such as a 10-km competitive runner who completes a 10-km time trial in practice. In these cases, athletes can use this as an opportunity to practice their specific nutrition strategies they plan to use on race day. This runner may eat the pre-event meal during training that she plans to eat on race day, as well as practice her during-race nutrition strategies she will use during competition. If she plans on drinking 4 oz of sports drink at the halfway point during the race, she should practice this in training. Other athletes may compete in events they do not actually complete in training, including some ultraendurance races, though these athletes can use their long training day to best approximate race day nutrition strategies.

Athletes should attempt to mimic race day conditions when possible. If the race is at 7 a.m., a cyclist who has a weekly "long ride" approaching the distance of the race should train early in the morning as well. This allows for practicing pre-event meals that best simulate race condition. If the event will be at a higher altitude, athletes should try and train at higher altitudes when possible. Environmental conditions can have a significant impact on tolerance for nutrition practices, as the more the body can adapt to these conditions, the more likely it is that race day will go smoothly.

Logistical concerns should be factored in as well. If athletes will need shuttling to the race start, this should be considered in advance so that prerace nutrition can be planned accordingly. If the race will provide aid stations or other forms of support, athletes should find out the details in advance. Athletes should inquire if there will be aid stations and, if so, what products they will be providing. If an aid station will be providing one brand of sport gels, for example, an athlete may want to consider training with that brand of gel, or finding a way to carry their own supplies. Different sports nutrition products have different ingredients, and race day is not the time to discover an athlete experiences gastrointestinal distress with specific ingredients. Will aid stations or race support allow drop-offs where athletes can drop their own nutrition supplies ahead of time? These are all important considerations.

An athlete should be as prepared as possible for race day. Pre-event meal, the night before or the morning of or both, should be finalized ahead of time and practiced more than once. This may require packing the meal with them if the athlete is traveling for an event, or knowing what foods will be available at the destination and practicing with those foods. Any products of fluids to be consumed during the event should be purchased, or planned for, ahead of time. Even recovery nutrition should be factored in. Foods that meet the athlete's recovery needs should be packed if it is known that food will not otherwise be available after competition. Every detail of race day nutrition should be thought through and planned for.

Definition

Nutrient density—the nutrient content of a food in proportion to the calories it contains.

References

American College of Sports Medicine, M.N. Sawka, L.M. Burke, E.R. Eichner, R.J. Maughan, S.J. Montain, and N.S. Stachenfeld. 2007. "American College of Sports Medicine Position Stand. Exercise and Fluid Replacement." *Medicine and Science in Sports and Exercise* 39, no. 2, pp. 377–90. doi:10.1249/mss.0b013e31802ca597

Arnall, D.A., A.G. Nelson, J. Quigley, S. Lex, T. Dehart, and P. Fortune. 2007. "Supercompensated Glycogen Loads Persist 5 Days in Resting Trained Cyclists." *European Journal of Applied Physiology* 99, no. 3, pp. 251–56. doi:10.1007/s00421-006-0340-4

Barnes, M.J. 2014. "Alcohol: Impact on Sports Performance and Recovery in Male Athletes." *Sports Medicine* 44, no. 7, pp. 909–19. doi:10.1007/s40279-014-0192-8

Bergstrom, J., L. Hermansen, E. Hultman, and B. Saltin. 1967. "Diet, Muscle Glycogen and Physical Performance." *Acta Physiologica Scandinavica* 71, no. 2, pp. 140–50. doi:10.1111/j.1748-1716.1967.tb03720.x

Burke, L.M., J.A. Hawley, S.H. Wong, and A.E. Jeukendrup. 2011. "Carbohydrates for Training and Competition." *Journal of Sports Sciences* 29, Suppl 1, pp. S17–27. doi:10.1080/02640414.2011.585473

Bussau, V.A., T.J. Fairchild, A. Rao, P. Steele, and P.A. Fournier. 2002. "Carbohydrate Loading in Human Muscle: An Improved 1 Day Protocol." *European Journal of Applied Physiology* 87, no. 3, pp. 290–95. doi:10.1007/s00421-002-0621-5

Fairchild, T.J., S. Fletcher, P. Steele, C. Goodman, B. Dawson, and P.A. Fournier. 2002. "Rapid Carbohydrate Loading After a Short Bout of Near Maximal-Intensity Exercise." *Medicine and Science in Sports and Exercise* 34, no. 6, pp. 980–86. doi:10.1097/00005768-200206000-00012

Ford, J.A. 2007. "Alcohol Use Among College Students: A Comparison of Athletes and Nonathletes." *Substance Use and Misuse* 42, no. 9, pp. 1367–77. doi:10.1080/10826080701212402

Goforth, H.W., Jr., D. Laurent, W.K. Prusaczyk, K.E. Schneider, K.F. Petersen, and G.I. Shulman. 2003. "Effects of Depletion Exercise and Light Training on Muscle Glycogen Supercompensation in Men." *American Journal of Physiology Endocrinology and Metabolism* 285, no. 6, pp. E1304–11. doi:10.1152/ajpendo.00209.2003

Havemann, L., and J.H. Goedecke. 2008. "Nutritional Practices of Male Cyclists Before and During an Ultraendurance Event." *International Journal of Sport Nutrition and Exercise Metabolism* 18, no. 6, pp. 551–66.

Heaney, S., H. O'Connor, G. Naughton, and J. Gifford. 2008. "Towards an Understanding of the Barriers to Good Nutrition for Elite Athletes." *International Journal of Sports Science & Coaching* 3, no. 3, pp. 391–401. doi:10.1260/174795408786238542

Sedlock, D.A. 2008. "The Latest on Carbohydrate Loading: A Practical Approach." *Current Sports Medicine Reports* 7, no. 4. pp. 209–13. doi:10.1249/JSR.0b013e31817ef9cb

Sherman, W.M., D.L. Costill, W.J. Fink, and J.M. Miller. 1981. "Effect of Exercise-Diet Manipulation on Muscle Glycogen and Its Subsequent Utilization During Performance." *International Journal of Sports Medicine* 2, no. 2, pp. 114–18. doi:10.1055/s-2008-1034594

U.S. Department of Health and Human Services, U.S. Department of Agriculture, and U.S. Dietary Guidelines Advisory Committee. 2010. *Dietary Guidelines for Americans, 2010.* 7th ed. Washington, DC: G.P.O., HHS Publication.

CHAPTER 7

Foods First, Supplements Second

The concept of foods first, supplements second implies that individuals, including athletes, can meet most if not all of their nutrient needs through foods and typically do not require additional supplementation. Of course, there are circumstances where vitamin or mineral supplementation may be warranted such as in the case of diagnosed nutrient deficiencies or certain medical conditions. Overall, though, selecting nutrient-dense foods and following the principles of balance, variety, and moderation will result in an adequate intake (AI) of nutrients needed for health and performance. The concept of foods first, supplements second does allow for use of nutrition supplements by athletes for performance, such as sport nutrition products, but these sources of nutrients should be *supplemental*, that is, complement the nutrients from food forms and should not be relied upon as a primary nutrient source.

Athletes should be aware of the limited benefits from consuming dietary supplements. Even among the few dietary supplements that actually have substantial evidence supporting their efficacy, the margin of benefit is relatively small. This is in contrast to the numerous research studies that highlight the significant health and performance benefits resulting from a well-balanced diet, eaten at the appropriate time. Optimal nutrition habits can dramatically impact performance, while most peer-reviewed research indicates that dietary supplements have minimal ergogenic effects. Thus, for the athlete looking for a "quick fix," they should be aware that legal dietary supplements will not dramatically alter their exercise performance, and that investment in a sound nutrition plan is money well spent and more likely to support and even improve training capacity. Furthermore, a poor diet cannot be compensated for by using dietary supplements.

This section will examine supplement use by athletes. First, information will be provided on dietary supplements and how they are regulated in the United States, including information on the health and safety risks of using dietary supplements and strategies for minimizing these risks. This section will then present information on dietary supplements that are used on a daily basis for health and immune function as well as to meet nutrient needs. Finally, common supplements used for ergogenic purposes will be addressed.

An Overview of Dietary Supplements

Regulation of Dietary Supplements

In 1994, the United States Congress passed DSHEA—the Dietary Supplement Health and Education Act—that has significantly impacted the manufacturing and marketing of dietary supplements. DSHEA defines a dietary supplement as a product, other than tobacco, intended to supplement the diet and containing one or more of the following ingredients: vitamin, mineral, herb or botanical, amino acid, dietary substance to supplement the diet by increasing the total dietary intake, concentrate, metabolite, constituent extract, or a combination of any of the aforementioned ingredients. This act classifies dietary supplements as "foods," therefore they are not regulated the same as prescription and over-the-counter medications. According to DSHEA, supplement manufacturers do not need to provide evidence of the safety or efficacy of their products; rather, it is up to the U.S. Food and Drug Administration (FDA) to prove a supplement is harmful. Because of limited resources of the FDA, as well as the thousands of supplement products available on the market, there is very little oversight of supplement products. Supplement makers are supposed to follow good manufacturing practices, which include ensuring products contain what is documented on the label. However, little is done to ensure this is actually the case.

The outcome of DSHEA is that dietary supplements are poorly regulated in the United States, as they are in most countries. This can result in statements being made on supplement labels (such as "Supports metabolism...") that have not been substantiated. These structure function claims are legal but can be quite misleading for consumers because the word "supports" can often be misinterpreted as fact. Additionally, dietary supplements do not always contain what they say they do, and may contain ingredients that are not listed on the ingredient list. When herbal supplements have been analyzed for their contents, some products have been found to have potentially dangerous levels of arsenic, lead, mercury, and pesticide residues; this could have harmful effects on an athlete's health (U.S. Government Accountability Office 2010). There have been similar studies finding high levels of arsenic, cadmium, lead, and mercury in protein drinks (ConsumerReports 2012). Other reports have shown contaminants such as allergens or microbial contamination that could pose significant adverse health effects.

In addition to health consequences, dietary supplements may contain illegal or banned substances that would result in penalties for the athlete or being excluded from sport participation. In a study conducted by the International Olympic Committee examining nonhormonal muscle-building supplements, 18.8 percent of products purchased from the United States contained banned substances (Geyer et al. 2004). In these cases, athletes may assume they are taking a safe and effective product when, in reality, they are risking a positive drug test that would get them banned from the competition.

Another risk of dietary supplements is that they may not contain the ingredients that are listed. In fact, some supplements may only contain a fraction of the active ingredient consumers believe that they are taking. An athlete may believe they are taking a supplement containing creatine, for example, when in reality there is very little creatine contained in the product. Thus, due to poor oversight over the supplement industry as a whole, the purity of a supplement should never be assumed.

Supplement Use Among Athletes

Nutrition supplements are concentrated sources of nutrients and other substances that have a nutritional or physiological effect on the body. Nutrition supplements are distinct from illicit drugs, which are substances banned by the World Anti-Doping Agency (WADA), a governing body that regulates substances for Olympic Athletes. Additionally, various professional and amateur sports governing bodies, such as US Soccer, USA Track & Field, USA Wrestling, and others, provide regulations specific to their sports. Collegiate athletes fall under the auspices of the National Collegiate Athletic Association (NCAA), which has its own list of banned substances. See Table 7.1.

Depending on how supplements are defined, reports of supplement use among athletes vary widely. In a study of elite Canadian athletes (Erdman et al. 2007), supplement use has been reported as high as 90 percent, while significantly lower intakes have been reported in other populations, such as a report of supplement use by 28 percent of Brazilian runners (Salgado et al. 2014). Among different population of athletes, rate of supplement use, as well as type of supplements used will vary according to the level of play and desired physical attributes associated with success. In general, elite-level athletes tend to have a higher reported use of supplements than recreational athletes. Younger athletes generally have a lower reported usage than older athletes, though younger athletes participating at the elite level report higher consumption of supplements (Dietz et al. 2014). Women are more likely to use supplements to address nutrient or medical deficiencies (real or perceived), whereas males are more likely to seek out supplement usage for strength, speed, and performance gains (Erdman et al. 2007). Further, individual sport athletes are more likely to use supplements than team sport athletes (Giannopoulou et al. 2013).

Table 7.1 Banned substances by the WADA & NCAA

Substances banned by the WADA	Substances banned by the NCAA
Anabolic androgenic steroids	Stimulants
Growth factors (human growth hormone)	Anabolic agents
Beta-2-agnosists (albuterol)	Alcohol and beta blockers (for rifle only)
Stimulants (amphetamines)	Diuretics and other masking agents
Diuretics (Lasix)	Street drugs
Narcotics	Peptide hormones and analogues
Beta blockers	Anti-estrogens
Glucocorticoids	Beta-2 agonists
Cannabinoid	
Erythropoietin	

The most commonly reported supplements used are sports drinks, sports bars, multivitamins and minerals, protein supplements, and vitamin C. These supplements and others that athletes consume will be examined later in this chapter; with the exception of sports drinks and sports bars, as these have been discussed in Chapter 4. Energy drinks are another popular product that falls under the category of dietary supplements, and given their popularity among younger athletes, these will be highlighted in "Practical Applications" at the end of this chapter.

There are many reasons athletes choose to take dietary supplements. Supplements may be taken to improve overall health and to optimize immune function or they may be taken to address nutrient deficiencies, whether real or perceived. Additionally, many athletes seek a competitive edge and seek supplements to improve strength, speed, endurance, or decrease recovery time. There are athletes who feel pressure to take supplements because of marketing schemes, such as the use of professional athlete testimonials. A sport nutrition professional should be aware of supplements that are being taken by an athlete, why they are taking them, the brand and dose being consumed, and length of consumption. The more the practitioner understands about an athlete's supplement use, the better they can guide the athlete on appropriate and safe consumption of these products.

A good practitioner needs to have at least a basic understanding of the current state of sports nutrition supplement research. The nutrition professional who rejects the use of all supplements may be dismissed by athletes who are seeking credible information. Rather, sports nutrition practitioners should provide unbiased, research-based information to athletes regarding supplement use. Ultimately, it is the decision of the athlete as to whether or not a supplement is appropriate for them and worth the money as well as any potential risks, but athletes can only make informed decisions when given access to credible resources.

A significant concern with supplement use is that many athletes (up to 85 percent of supplements users in one study) report to have very little knowledge of side effects of the supplements, including potential health concerns and possible negative nutrient interactions (Dietz et al. 2014; Erdman et al. 2007). Athletes are generally unaware that the supplements that they are taking may contain more or less or different ingredients than what is listed on the label, not to mention potential contamination with illegal substances or other contaminants. These risks illustrate the importance of educating athletes on supplement use by a sports nutrition professional.

Supplements Taken by Athletes

Supplements Used to Meet Nutrient Needs

Multivitamins

Multivitamin use is one of the most commonly reported nutrition supplements used by athletes. Multivitamins typically contain most if not all essential vitamins and minerals including many trace minerals. Athletes take multivitamins to improve health and increase resistance to illness and disease, as well as to improve physical performance. However, there is no research to substantiate that taking a multivitamin provides any of the aforementioned benefits and a nutrient-dense diet that is characterized by balance, variety, and moderation is more than likely to contain all the vitamins and minerals in necessary quantities. An athlete would only need a multivitamin if they are not able to meet their nutrient needs through food or if they are prone to nutrient deficiencies such as anemia. Exceptions that warrant multivitamin use include: athletes who eliminate certain food groups from their diets, such as vegans who do not consume animal products (to be discussed in Chapter 8), or individuals who eat very few fruits and vegetables. Some athletes risk low calcium or vitamin D intake, which will be addressed in the following chapter. Other athletes in specific stages of the lifecycle, such as a pregnant woman who exercises, may also warrant taking a prenatal multivitamin to meet her increased nutrient needs. Athletes with a restrictive intake in efforts to alter body composition may benefit from a multivitamin as well. The nutrition professional who conducts a nutrition assessment of the daily diet of an athlete will be able to identify any key nutrients that risk inadequate intake. Foods should be targeted to meet these needs when possible, and supplements can "fill the gap" if these efforts are not successful.

One challenge with multivitamins is that there is no standardized quantity of each nutrient that a multivitamin should contain. This results in significant variability in the amounts of nutrients between products. For example, one multivitamin may contain 100 percent of the Recommended Dietary Allowance (RDA) or AI for each vitamin and mineral, while another product may have 50 percent of the RDA for calcium, or 5,000 percent of vitamin E. The RDA is the average daily intake of a nutrient that is sufficient to meet the nutrient needs for 98 percent of the healthy population. A common misconception, however, that if some is good, more is better. If 100 percent of vitamin B6 is sufficient, then 200 percent must be better. This is simply not the case. In most cases, 100 percent of a nutrient is all one needs.

Taking a multivitamin may not be harmful per se, especially if the multivitamin they are taking is moderate in the amounts of vitamins and minerals it contains (such as 50 to 100 percent of the RDA). Multivitamins that contain excessive amounts of nutrients, however, may risk reaching toxic levels especially if individuals are consuming additional amounts of nutrients from food sources. Additionally, many cereals, sports bars, sports drinks, and other products are often formulated with added vitamins and minerals and so an athlete may be getting much more than they realize. There are other risks of excessive consumption of certain nutrients that are outside of the scope of this text. In general, athletes should be encouraged to meet their nutrient needs from food sources and can avoid the added expense of a multivitamin unless dietary analysis reflects a nutrient-poor diet.

Single Vitamin and Mineral Supplements

Some athletes take a supplement containing a singular nutrient, such as calcium, vitamin C, vitamin E, or iron. Athletes requiring calcium or iron supplementation will be addressed in Chapter 8. In general, the same principle applied to multivitamins applies to single vitamin use. Most athletes can meet their needs for these nutrients through food sources and do not require additional supplementation.

Antioxidants. Exhaustive exercise increases the body's exposure to free radicals, which are highly reactive substances that damage cellular DNA and cell membranes. Free radicals cause oxidative stress on muscles and other tissues, resulting in oxidative damage. Antioxidants, including vitamin A, C, and E, are molecules that can neutralize these free radicals before they cause harm. Thus, it has been suggested by some that athletes should supplement with high doses of vitamins A, C, and E to reduce oxidative stress, protect the muscle from oxidative damage, thus improving exercise performance (Nikolaidis et al. 2012).While there is some research supporting reduced oxidative stress and muscle damage postexercise with vitamin A, C, and E supplementation, there is also evidence suggesting that reducing the free radical load blocks essential physiological adaptations to training. It has been shown that through exposure to free radicals produced from exercise, the body upregulates its own antioxidant response; taking antioxidant supplementation may blunt this response and may even have a pro-oxidant effect. In fact, one recent study looking at endurance athletes found that those taking an antioxidant supplement reduced improvements in VO_2 max, compared to the placebo group, supporting the belief that antioxidants may impede training adaptations (Skaug, Sveen, and Raastad 2013). At this time, the research is inconclusive and thus it is not recommend that athletes take high doses of antioxidants, particularly vitamins C and E, until more convincing evidence is available. Rather, athletes should be encouraged to consume more dietary sources of antioxidants, especially from food sources such as fruits and vegetables.

Protein Supplements

Protein supplements are some of the most commonly reported supplements taken by athletes. Common reasons for protein supplement use include seeking increased muscle mass, as well as improved performance and recovery from exercise. As a brief review from information previously presented in Chapter 4, in order to increase muscle mass, amino acids are needed in sufficient quantity to stimulate muscle protein synthesis. Specifically, indispensable amino acids and particularly the branched-chain amino acids (leucine, isoleucine, and valine) are required for muscle protein synthesis. Leucine especially has been shown to be important in the signaling cascade that promotes muscle protein synthesis. The current recommendation based on the majority of research findings is to consume 20 to 25 g of high-quality protein as soon as possible after exercise.

Athletes can meet these recommendations through either traditional foods or protein supplements, as one is no "better" than the other. What must be considered is the *quality* of the protein in the food or supplement. For example, when comparing protein supplements, the most commonly marketed, used, and researched forms of protein found in these supplements are whey, casein, and soy proteins. Each has a favorable indispensable amino acid profile, but studies comparing these three protein forms and their effect on muscle protein synthesis have consistently shown that whey protein stimulates greater muscle protein synthesis compared with comparable amounts of casein and soy (Phillips et al. 2012). The exact mechanism for this difference is unknown, but is probably due to the high content of leucine, which is known to stimulate muscle protein synthesis. On a practical note, milk is also a good source of whey protein as well as carbohydrates so it may be an optimal "protein supplement" that is also affordable.

Few studies have compared food forms of protein with supplemental forms regarding how athletes meet their protein needs. A recent study conducted by Burke et al. in 2012 measured postprandial plasma amino acid levels 1 hour after consuming 20 g of various sources of protein (eggs, meat, and milk that were consumed independently) and compared them to a liquid meal supplement containing protein (PowerBar Protein Plus™ containing a trisource mixture of 1:1:1 whey, casein, and soy protein). The results showed that while the total amino acid delivery in the plasma was similar among the different protein types, liquid forms of protein reached peak concentrations twice as quickly as food forms; additionally, milk reached a statistically significant faster peak leucine concentration when compared to meat, eggs, or the protein supplement food forms as well as the protein-containing supplement (Burke et al. 2012).

To date, there is little evidence to suggest that protein supplements provide an additional ergogenic benefit when compared to food-based sources of protein. What remain the most important factors are the quantity, quality, and timing of protein intake postexercise.

Other important considerations when helping athletes meet their protein needs are convenience and cost. Convenience is one factor that can significantly impact an athlete's ability to meet their nutrient needs. Protein supplements can be easily packed and taken with athletes for postexercise consumption. This is important to many athletes but there are also many forms of portable foods that contain protein. Cost is another factor when assessing if protein supplements are appropriate as many protein supplements can be quite costly and the cost per serving can be significantly more than food forms, such as a glass of milk. Milk provides a high-quality form of protein; it also provides calcium, vitamin D, potassium, vitamin A, and vitamin K. Protein supplements may have added vitamins and minerals, though the bioavailability of added nutrients is typically less than that of natural food forms, which should be calculated into the financial assessment. Athletes should also be advised that protein supplements and other muscle-building supplements are generally those that are at the greatest risk of being contaminated with anabolic steroids or other substances.

Supplements Taken for Performance-Enhancing Effects

While overall health is one reason athletes take nutrition supplements, achieving performance benefits is another frequently cited motivation. Athletes are motivated to increase muscle mass, boost aerobic and anaerobic capacity, and improve recovery. As a consequence, athletes may seek any competitive edge they can find. In addition to training and nutrition practices, athletes turn to **ergogenic aids** to give them an advantage over their opponents and for personal improvement. Following are some of the most commonly sought out ergogenic aids that have at least minimal research to indicate if there is a potential benefit, though this is by no means an exhaustive list. Because sports nutrition products and ergogenic aids are continuously being developed and researched, the sports nutrition practitioner needs to stay on top of current research to ensure appropriate recommendations are provided.

Caffeine

Caffeine is the most common psychostimulant taken worldwide. It is not currently a banned substance in sports, though for many years high amounts detected in the urine were considered illegal according to the WADA; the exception is that for NCAA athletes, urinary caffeine levels exceeding 15 mcg/dL could result in a banned substance test, though this amount would be difficult to achieve with food and drinks alone. Caffeine has been shown in numerous research studies to improve endurance capacity as well as power output in submaximal and high-intensity exercise when taken before or during exercise (Hodgson, Randell, and Jeukendrup 2013). Initially, the performance benefit of caffeine was thought to be the result of increased fat oxidation through action on the sympathetic nervous system, thus exerting a glycogen-sparing effect. This theory has been refuted in light of more substantial research demonstrating caffeine's performance-enhancing effect by acting on the peripheral and central nervous system. Specifically, caffeine lowers perception of pain and exertion, allowing athletes to work harder, as well as improving motor recruitment and supporting muscle contraction. Indeed, in various time trial studies, athletes' performance was improved when consuming caffeine (Desbrow et al. 2012; Irwin et al. 2011).

Since the establishment of caffeine as an ergogenic aid, research has investigated questions regarding the optimal amount, timing, and form of caffeine consumed for performance benefit. Regarding dosing, it appears that 3 mg of caffeine per kg of body weight (3 mg/kg) produces an ergogenic effect with no additional benefits at greater amounts (Desbrow et al. 2012). For a 70-kg male, this equals 210 mg, or the amount of caffeine in a large cup of coffee. See Table 7.2. Amounts greater than 3 mg/kg increases the potential for negative side effects including: increased heart rate and blood pressure due to higher catecholamine levels resulting from caffeine intake, higher blood lactate levels, gastrointestinal distress, nervousness, shakiness, mental confusion, and an inability to focus. These adverse effects could be debilitating in an athletic environment, so taking the lowest dose needed to receive a performance benefit is a prudent approach.

Caffeine peaks in the blood between 30 and 90 minutes after ingestion and has a half-life of around 5 hours. Thus, consuming caffeine approximately 1 hour before exercise helps to ensure optimal levels of caffeine in the blood. For long endurance events, there may be a performance benefit to consuming caffeine late in the exercise bout. Endurance athletes may want to consider including caffeinated products, which include some sports drinks, gels, and bars, in the second half of a race but only after experimenting with these products in training (Cox et al. 2002).

Table 7.2 Caffeine content in common foods

Food or drink	Serving size	Caffeine (mg)
Coffee house brewed coffee	16 oz	330
Coffee house café latte	16 oz	150
Single Espresso	1 shot	75
Coffee house iced coffee	16 oz	165
Home brewed coffee	2 tbsp/12 oz	100–160
Home brewed instant coffee	2 tbsp/12 oz	148
Coffee house decaf coffee	16 oz	15–25
Black tea, brewed 3 minutes	8 oz	30–80
Green tea, brewed 3 minutes	8 oz	35–60
Herbal tea, brewed	8 oz	0
Most colas, diet or regular	12 oz	35–47
Mountain Dew™, diet or regular	12 oz	54
Most energy drinks	16 oz	160–200
Jelly Belly Extreme Sport Beans™	1 package/1 oz	50
Clif Shot Bloks™ with caffeine	3 pieces/1/2 package	50
Gu's and gels with caffeine	1 packet	20–30
Excedrin Migraine™	2 tablets	130
Caffeine powder	200 mg	200
Liquid caffeine	½ teaspoon	41.5

Source: Center for Science in the Public Interest (2012) and manufacturers' websites, http://www.cspinet.org/new/cafchart.htm

The form of caffeine delivery may also have ergogenic relevance. Specifically, it has been questioned if coffee provides an additional ergogenic benefit over caffeinated sports products or caffeine pills. Most studies, though not all, show a performance benefit when coffee is consumed as the source of caffeine. Studies that do not show a benefit of coffee as the source of caffeine may have flawed methodologies that include using time to exhaustion test to assess performance (Graham, Hibbert, and Sathasivam 1998). This can be a less valid, or realistic, way to assess performance in athletes since most forms of competition are assessing speed or other variables, not the time until the athlete is exhausted. Conversely, a more recent study compared the same amount of caffeine in coffee compared to caffeine supplements using more realistic measures of performance (a time trial) and found that both products had comparable performance benefits (Hodgson, Randell, and Jeukendrup 2013). This study may be a better representative of the scenarios an athlete faces.

There are other considerations when examining the ergogenic potential of caffeine. There has been some question as to whether or not habitual users receive the same benefit from caffeine as those who abstain from caffeine for a period of time, then prior to competition, consume caffeine. However, research indicates that caffeine abstinence does not seem to be necessary and performance is benefited equally in habitual versus nonhabitual users (Irwin et al. 2011).

All in all, caffeine is supported by the research as an ergogenic aid for submaximal and endurance exercise; there does not appear to be a benefit for single-effort strength or power efforts. Three mg/kg appears to be a safe and effective dose to be taken 60 minutes before exercise with benefit to endurance athletes consuming caffeine late in exercise (about 3 mg/kg as well). Athletes should experiment with caffeine consumption well before an athletic competition to have a thorough understanding of how their body responds to caffeine consumption during exercise. This will help to develop the most effective strategy for optimal performance.

Creatine

Creatine is another dietary supplement that has been well studied in the field of exercise and sports science. Creatine is an amino acid derivative that is naturally produced in the body by the kidneys, in the amount of about 1 to 2 g/day, with additional 1 to 2 g/day consumed from food sources, especially meat and fish. Ninety-five percent of the body's creatine is stored in the muscle, which highlights the important function of creatine, previously discussed in Chapter 3. Chapter 3 also discusses the role of phosphocreatine in regenerating adenine triphosphate (ATP) from ADP and is the primary energy source in the first several seconds of high-intensity exercise; creatine is a required component of this molecule. Consequently, supplementation with creatine in conjunction with resistance training has been shown to increase strength performance by increasing the total creatine pool, regenerating ATP more rapidly in between resistance training sets, thus allowing the athlete to train at a higher intensity. This results in greater strength, power, and fat-free mass gains in athletes. Creatine plays a role in improving muscle damage following exercise, thus attenuating a loss in strength.

Creatine has been shown to enhance short-duration, high-intensity exercise through rapid energy provision as well as improved calcium reuptake in the muscle cell. Creatine can also increase muscle glycogen stores when combined with a high carbohydrate diet for high-intensity or long-duration glycogen-depleting exercise, yet the increase in body mass resulting from water retention may negate this benefit because the athlete has more mass to carry. There is limited data to suggest creatine may improve endurance exercise and more research is needed to support this claim. In general, though, it appears that an increased creatine pool from supplementation supports favorable physiological adaptations from aerobic exercise, including increased plasma volume and ventilatory threshold with reduced oxygen consumption in submaximal exercise (Cooper et al. 2012). Additionally, on a more functional level, a recent meta-analysis supported the role creatine in delaying age-related muscle loss, or *sarcopenia*, preserving strength, and maintaining functional performance (Devries and Phillips 2014) in older individuals. This addresses a significant health concern related to the aging process.

Because creatine is a naturally occurring substance both produced endogenously and consumed from food sources, it is not a banned substance on any doping list. Creatine appears to be relatively safe. The most common adverse effect experienced by athletes is transient water retention of up to 1.5 kg in males (or up to 750 g in women), though this typically resolves after about a week (Mihic et al. 2000). There have been concerns that creatine may harm renal function, and while no consistent human research has been able to identify this (only single cases have been documented), it is recommended that those individuals with impaired renal functioning or who have renal disease, or those who are predisposed to such, should avoid creatine supplementation.

The side effects of supplementation have been studied for up to 4 years without any apparent adverse effects, though consumption of creatine for periods longer than that has not been studied and so long-term safety cannot be established. Contrary to initial belief, creatine does not appear to cause dehydration (Cooper et al. 2012). Gastrointestinal distress has been reported in about five percent of athletes, though it seems in these cases the supplement was not mixed properly or was taken on an empty stomach; thus, ensuring proper mixing of the supplement and taking it with food could alleviate these issues (Tarnopolsky 2010).

A typical creatine supplementation protocol includes a loading phase and then a maintenance phase. The loading phase includes consuming 20 to 25g of creatine monohydrate split into 4 to 5 daily intakes of 5 g each for 5 days for optimal creatine retention. A more recent protocol of consuming 20 g/day for 5 days but splitting the dosage up into 1 g every 30 minutes may maximize creatine stores, though the practicality of consuming a supplement every 30 minutes has to be considered. This is followed by a maintenance phase of consuming 3 to 5g/day of creatine monohydrate to sustain muscle creatine stores. It is important to note some individuals appear to respond more positively to creatine supplementation than others, that is, there seem to be responders versus nonresponders, which seems to be mediated by initial creatine and type II muscle fiber content. Additionally, an individual's response may be based upon typical dietary intake; those who have a high dietary intake of creatine from animal products may be less able to increase their storage. Vegetarian athletes, on the other hand, who are more likely to have a lower dietary intake of creatine may see increased muscle creatine stores from supplementation. Women, in general, tend to respond less to creatine supplementation than do men. Individuals will only know if they are responders through trial and error but should be aware they may not actually respond significantly to supplementation.

There are different forms of creatine supplementation. Creatine monohydrate is the most extensively studied form. Some recent research supports potentially greater creatine storage with creatine salts, such as creatine pyruvate, creatine citrate, or creatine malate, especially when these types are consumed with carbohydrate. However, more research is needed to explore this. In general, there seems to be 25 percent greater creatine retention when consumed with carbohydrate or protein or both for all forms of creatine which is mediated by the simultaneous release of insulin (Cooper et al. 2012).

Overall, creatine appears to be a safe and efficacious supplement to increase strength, muscle mass, and performance in short-duration, high-intensity sport, as well as improve aerobic capacity. Supplementation should follow established protocols, and forthcoming research may provide additional recommendations for other forms of creatine. Intake should not exceed recommended doses. If an athlete has any concern about the safety of creatine supplementation, a urinary albumin-excretion rate can be used to assess kidney functioning and is relatively easy and inexpensive. Individuals should monitor their own response to determine if they are indeed benefiting from supplementation. As with all supplements, great care should be taken to ensure the purity of the supplement. More on this will be discussed at the conclusion of the chapter. Additionally, while creatine use can be common among adolescent athletes, given that the long-term safety is unknown, and that it is not a regulated substance, many health professionals believe adolescent athletes should not use creatine supplements.

Buffering Agents: Sodium Bicarbonate and Beta Alanine

For a long time it was thought that fatigue during high-intensity exercise relying largely upon anaerobic glycolysis was due to the accumulation of lactate. However, it is now accepted that fatigue in this context is primarily due to a decrease in pH resulting from hydrogen ion (H+) accumulation from working muscle, a phenomenon known as metabolic acidosis. In fact, while optimal blood pH is 7.4, during exercise this can decrease to 7.1, with muscle pH going as low as 6.8. Consequently, an alkalizing agent that could buffer the blood would attenuate the onset of fatigue and allow continued provision of energy through anaerobic glycolysis. Two of these buffers have been well researched and demonstrate promising results.

Sodium bicarbonate. Sodium bicarbonate has been studied for over 80 years for its performance effects in strength sports. Sodium bicarbonate increases the availability of bicarbonate in the blood, allowing it to accept a hydrogen ion to form carbonic acid; from there, carbonic acid is dissociated and carbon dioxide is excreted by the lung through respiration (see Figure 7.1). In fact, most but not all research examining the effects of sodium bicarbonate supplementation has found that performance is enhanced in events of high power output lasting 1 to 7 minutes; this includes sports such as middle-distance swimming, middle-distance running, and rowing. Additionally, longer sports that have intermittent

$$H^+ + HCO_3 \leftrightarrow H_2CO_3 \leftrightarrow CO_2 + H_2O$$

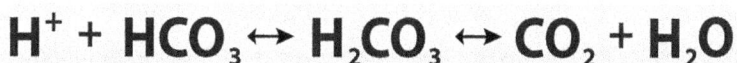

Sodium bicarbonate combines with hydrogen ions produced during high intensity exercise yielding carbonic acid, which dissociates into carbon dioxide and water to help buffer the pH of the blood.

Figure 7.1 Sodium bicarbonate

or sustained high-intensity output have seen ergogenic benefits as well, including team sports such as soccer, basketball, racquet sports, and even combative sports (Burke 2013). Training and competition that includes repeated sprints see improvements in performance, especially in subsequent bouts or sprints, since sodium bicarbonate's mechanism of action is on the recovery of acid–base balance in between efforts. Research has shown that the size of effect, or the magnitude of benefit, is greatest in untrained athletes, though even a small benefit among elite-level athletes can make the difference between first and fourth place (Peart, Siegler, and Vince 2012).

A common challenge with sodium bicarbonate consumption are gastrointestinal side effects that athletes experience when supplementing with this product, including stomach pain, nausea, diarrhea, and vomiting. Obviously, this can be quite disruptive to sport performance and could result in worsened outcomes. Athletes should always experiment with bicarbonate supplementation apart from competition to assess their own tolerance. While household sodium bicarbonate is the least expensive form of the product, there is some thought that this form results in the lowest tolerance. Thus, capsule form or taking a pharmaceutical powder in flavored liquids may help improve tolerance. The recommended dosage is 300 mg per kg of body weight (300 mg/kg), and should be taken 1 to 2 hours before the event for optimal alkalizing of the blood. Future research can help identify loading protocols within this time period that may minimize gastrointestinal distress.

Beta-alanine (β-alanine). β-Alanine is another supplement being investigated for its potential to serve as a buffer during high-intensity exercise by increasing the efflux of hydrogen ions, though unlike sodium bicarbonate, β-alanine is an intracellular buffer. β-Alanine is actually the rate-limiting precursor to carnosine, a dipeptide found in abundant quantities in skeletal muscle. Some carnosine is synthesized in the muscle from dietary components, especially meat, though maximal muscle carnosine content cannot be achieved by this process alone since normal food sources do not provide adequate amounts of β-alanine. Thus, there have been some studies that have found with β-alanine supplementation that intracellular buffering capacity is increased and consequently so is exercise performance.

The exact sport types that might benefit from β-alanine supplementation are still being examined. The majority of research shows improved performance with high-intensity, high-power-output exercise lasting one to four, and up to seven minutes; there is the potential for enhanced sprint performance at the end of a longer-distance event, though studies are mixed on this (Bellinger 2014; Blancquaert, Everaert, and Derave 2015). Not only may β-alanine supplementation improve competitive performance, but also there is a reason to believe it may also allow athletes to train at higher intensities for longer periods, thus increasing their overall exercise capacity.

While the research is clear that supplementation augments carnosine concentration, this may or may not translate to performance benefits. Many but not all studies have shown an ergogenic effect of β-alanine supplementation in high-intensity events; consequently, an athlete considering β-alanine should gauge their own performance in assessing if they are indeed receiving benefits. Some studies have shown trained athletes may see smaller performance gains than untrained individuals, though this small increase in performance can be meaningful to elite-level athletes where finishing times can be within milliseconds of each other.

There are no standard protocols outlined for β-alanine supplementation. The most common approach seems to be to consume ~80 mg/kg/day. Athletes should not take more than 10 mg/kg at a time to avoid the potential for paresthesia, which includes a tingling or prickling ("pins and needles") sensation. Thus, smaller doses should be consumed throughout the day and taken with meals to maximize carnosine loading (Bellinger 2014).

In summary, there is promise for intracellular and extracellular buffers to mitigate the effects of metabolic acidosis thus delaying fatigue during high-intensity exercise, allowing athletes to train harder and improve competitive performance. Sodium bicarbonate has more substantial support for its efficacy, with β-alanine showing more mixed results. In either case, athletes considering these supplements should experiment with them according to the proposed protocols and assess their own performance to see if they are benefitting. More research is needed to identify standard dosages and protocols, especially with β-alanine to better understand which athletes may benefit the most. All athletes must assess if any potential side effects are worth the potential for improved performance benefit.

Other Supplements: Those Showing Promise and Those with Minimal Support

Table 7.3 lists other dietary supplements commonly taken by athletes. The table is divided into those that show promise for improving performance, and those that have limited support for their efficacy in performance enhancement. Because the research and development of dietary supplements is constantly changing, it is up to the athlete and sport nutrition practitioner to stay on top of the most current research to accurately translate recent findings.

Table 7.3 **Efficacy of common dietary supplements taken by athletes**

Supplements with promise for performance	Comments
Beetroot or nitrate	Has been studied in reference to improving cardiovascular health by increasing blood flow and reducing blood pressure; this may translate to improved oxygen utilization in athletes but more research is needed.
Branched-chain fatty acids	Do not appear to have a performance benefit, but may improve delayed-onset muscle soreness (DOMS) and fatigue after various types of workouts.
Probiotics	May improve immune health, particularly related to upper and lower respiratory infections to which endurance athletes may be more susceptible; shows promise in improving gastrointestinal issues in endurance athletes as well.

(Continued)

Table 7.3 Efficacy of common dietary supplements taken by athletes   (Continued)

Supplements with limited support for performance	Comments
β-hydroxy-β-methylbutyrate (HMB)	HMB shows mixed results in its application to high-intensity, strength-based training. Some studies do demonstrate improved recovery from muscle damage resulting from high-intensity strength training, and small increases in muscle hypertrophy have been seen in some individuals.
Ribose	Theoretically may improve ATP resynthesis and increase recovery from high-intensity training, though evidence insufficient to recommend supplementation at this point.
Vitamin E	See discussion earlier in chapter
Vitamin C	See discussion earlier in chapter
Quercetin	Quercetin has shown a small but positive effect on some, but not all, endurance athletes. This effect is potentially mediated through its effect on increasing oxidative capacity. More studies are needed.
Bovine colostrum	There has been limited research determining bovine colostrum's effect on potentially improving immune health and gastrointestinal integrity in endurance athletes; more research is needed to assess efficacy.
L-arginine	Limited research supports L-arginine's efficacy in increasing vasodilation via nitric oxide; research does not show strong support for L-arginine's role in increasing growth hormone secretion and consequent stimulation of protein synthesis.
Glutamine	Has very limited research supporting its efficacy in improving immune functioning, particularly upper respiratory tract infections. Still being investigated for its effects on immunodepression and other measures that could improve performance but so far very little evidence exists.

Medium chain triglycerides (MCT)	Does not show promise for improving exercise capacity by sparing glycogen through increased fat oxidation; MCTs do show promise in supporting weight loss through increased energy expenditure though more research is needed.
Carnitine	There is indirect support for carnitine's role in improving fat oxidation and sparing glycogen in endurance exercise, though currently there is no direct evidence that carnitine supplementation actually improves fat oxidation and improves performance.

Summary of Dietary Supplements and Athletes

Dietary supplements are popular among athletes and are consumed for a variety of reasons, though athletes should never assume supplements can replace proper nutrition practices. Due to poor regulation of supplements, individuals should be aware of the safety concerns as well as the efficacy of different products. Sports nutrition professionals should serve as a resource for current and unbiased dietary supplement information. Ultimately, athletes should be aware that the onus is on them to make a decision regarding dietary supplement use. Questions athletes can ask to guide their decision making are as follows:

- Is it safe?
- Is it pure?
- Is it effective?
- Is it illegal?
- Is it ethical?

Guiding athletes through these questions can provide a more complete picture for a cost–benefit analysis of supplement use and ultimately support athletes in achieving their optimal performance in a safe manner.

For additional resources, individuals can turn to the WADA, as well as the United States' committee, the U.S. Anti-Doping Agency (USADA).

Table 7.4 Resources for supplement evaluation

Safety resources	Purity resources	Purity and banned substances resources
MedWatch: www.fda.gov/ Safety/MedWatch/default.htm	U.S. Pharmacopeia Dietary Supplement Verification Program	NSF Certified for Sport
Quackwatch: http://quackwatch.org	ConsumerLab.com Quality Evaluation	Banned Substances Control Group partnered with Anti-Doping Research Laboratory
Website for Dietary Supplements **Certification Program**: www.nsf.org/services/ by-industry/dietary-supplements/ supplement-safety/	NSF International Dietary Supplements Certification Program	Informed Choice Program partnered with UK-based HFL Sport Science Testing Laboratory

Source: Additional resources for assessing dietary supplements' safety, purity, and content of banned substances. Modified from the National Athletic Trainers' Association Position Statement: Evaluation of Dietary Supplements for Performance Nutrition (Buell et al. 2013).

USADA has a "Supplement 411" on its website providing a great online educational tool for the risks and challenges of dietary supplement consumption. Table 7.4 provides additional resources on assessing products' safety, purity, and screening for banned substances.

Practical Applications: Are Energy Drinks Recommended for Athletes

Energy drinks are one of the most popular dietary supplements among adolescents, and energy drink manufacturers often market these products toward this population for their performance effects. Yet, energy drinks should not be confused for sports drinks, which are fluids designed to meet the hydration, electrolyte, and carbohydrate needs of athletes. Sports drinks have been formulated based upon extensive scientific studies designed to examine the optimal ratio of ingredients that will support optimal athletic performance. Energy drinks simply do not have the depth of research supporting them as do sports drinks.

While most sports drinks contain the appropriate concentration of carbohydrate for maximal absorption (6 to 8 percent carbohydrate), energy drinks often contain much higher concentrations of carbohydrates. The typical carbohydrate concentration is 11 to 12 percent, beyond the recommended upper range of 8 percent. Carbohydrate concentrations this high may result in delayed gastric emptying and gastrointestinal upset (Campbell et al. 2013). These beverages are also high in vitamins, minerals, caffeine, and other stimulants such as taurine, Guarana, amino acids, Ginkgo biloba, Carnitine, Green Tea, and many others. There is no empirical support that the addition of vitamins and minerals in the amounts contained in energy drinks provide a health benefit to the consumers. While some of the other added nutrients may have some support for an ergogenic effect on performance, such as the addition of β-alanine, these drinks typically do not contain the amounts of these nutrients that have been shown to have a performance benefit. Additionally, the manufacturers do not need to disclose how much of each herbal is contained in the drink if it is a "proprietary blend." Thus, an athlete may be getting a large dose of caffeine or other substance and not even realize it. This could have deleterious health and performance effects.

Energy drinks often make claims for improving alertness, energy metabolism, and performance in a whole host of sport settings, though their performance benefit is largely unsubstantiated. There have been some studies that indicate improved performance in mental focus, alertness, aerobic, and endurance performance, though the benefit seems largely to come from the addition of caffeine or carbohydrate or both; evidence for a benefit from the added stimulants is lacking. What is needed to provide greater support for energy drinks in sport contexts is to compare energy drinks with products containing the recommended amount of caffeine and carbohydrate that have already been established for performance enhancement. This would help avoid some of the potential negative side effects associated with energy drinks. So far this information is not available.

Some of the negative effects of energy drinks have to do with the caffeine content. Most energy drinks contain between 50 and 286 mg of caffeine (Torpy and Livingston 2013). While this amount appears to be safe, the actual amount is not regulated, which means the actual caffeine content could be quite variable among and between products.

Additionally, there is potential that other added stimulants, such as taurine, might have an additive effect with caffeine. Given that individuals may consume several servings of an energy drink, the risks of a high caffeine consumption become more likely, including tremors, insomnia, gastrointestinal distress, tachycardia, and more. Individuals with medical conditions including metabolic syndrome and diabetes should avoid energy drinks due to their high carbohydrate content and glycemic index, and individuals with cardiovascular disease may want to avoid these beverages as well given their cardiostimulant effects (Campbell et al. 2013). Additionally, there is concern regarding the use of energy drinks among adolescent athletes; these individuals have been seen to consume several of these products before, during, and after exercise and are experiencing dangerous tachycardia and cardiac events. The American Academy of Pediatrics (AAP) warns against the use of these products among individuals below 18 years of age.

Overall, educating an athlete who may consume energy drinks should include information on the pros and cons of these beverages. Energy drinks are not comparable to sports drinks, which have considerably more scientific support for their performance benefit. Some studies show some performance benefits of energy drinks, though much more is needed including short- and long-term studies. Because carbohydrate and caffeine are most likely the source of performance enhancement, athletes may want to consider safer methods for consuming these ingredients including products that have standardized amounts and less variability of ingredient quantities. Children and adolescent athletes should be cautioned against energy drink consumption because of a lack of research studies of the effects of these beverages on this population, especially on their growth and development. For athletes who do consume energy drinks it should be emphasized to avoid consuming large quantities given this is when adverse effects are most likely to occur.

If an athlete is motivated by performance, then they should choose products that have a proven performance benefit (i.e., sports drinks and regulated caffeine supplements) versus products with much less research and greater variability in its contents.

Definition

Ergogenic aids—a physical, mechanical, nutritional, psychological, or pharmacological technique or substance that has the potential to enhance performance.

References

Bellinger, P.M. 2014. "Beta-Alanine Supplementation for Athletic Performance: An Update." *Journal of Strength and Conditioning Research* 28, no. 6, pp. 1751–70. doi:10.1519/JSC.0000000000000327

Blancquaert, L., I. Everaert, and W. Derave. 2015. "Beta-Alanine Supplementation, Muscle Carnosine and Exercise Performance." *Current Opinion in Clinical Nutrition and Metabolic Care* 18, no. 1, pp. 63–70. doi:10.1097/MCO.0000000000000127

Buell, J.L., R. Franks, J. Ransone, M.E. Powers, K.M. Laquale, A. Carlson-Phillips, and Association National Athletic Trainers. 2013. "National Athletic Trainers' Association Position Statement: Evaluation of Dietary Supplements for Performance Nutrition." *Journal of Athletic Training* 48, no. 1, pp. 124–36. doi:10.4085/1062-6050-48.1.16

Burke, L.M. 2013. "Practical Considerations for Bicarbonate Loading and Sports Performance." *Nestle Nutrition Institute Workshop Series* 75, pp. 15–26. doi:10.1159/000345814

Burke, L.M., J.A. Winter, D. Cameron-Smith, M. Enslen, M. Farnfield, and J. Decombaz. 2012. "Effect of Intake of Different Dietary Protein Sources on Plasma Amino Acid Profiles at Rest and After Exercise." *International Journal of Sport Nutrition and Exercise Metabolism* 22, no. 6 , pp. 452–62.

Campbell, B., C. Wilborn, P. La Bounty, L. Taylor, M.T. Nelson, M. Greenwood, T.N. Ziegenfuss, H.L. Lopez, J.R. Hoffman, J.R. Stout, S. Schmitz, R. Collins, D.S. Kalman, J. Antonio, and R.B. Kreider. 2013. "International Society of Sports Nutrition Position Stand: Energy Drinks." *Journal of the International Society of Sports Nutrition* 10, no. 1, p. 1. doi:10.1186/1550-2783-10-1

ConsumerReports. 2012. "Protein Drinks." www.consumerreports.org/cro/2012/04/protein-drinks/index.htm (accessed November 26).

Cooper, R., F. Naclerio, J. Allgrove, and A. Jimenez. 2012. "Creatine Supplementation with Specific View to Exercise/Sports Performance: An Update." *Journal of the International Societyof Sports Nutrition* 9, no. 1, p. 33. doi:10.1186/1550-2783-9-33

Cox, G.R., B. Desbrow, P.G. Montgomery, M.E. Anderson, C.R. Bruce, T.A. Macrides, D.T. Martin, A. Moquin, A. Roberts, J.A. Hawley, and L.M. Burke. 2002. "Effect of Different Protocols of Caffeine Intake on Metabolism and Endurance Performance." *Journal of Applied Physiology* 93, no. 3, pp. 990–99. doi:10.1152/japplphysiol.00249.2002

Desbrow, B., C. Biddulph, B. Devlin, G.D. Grant, S. Anoopkumar-Dukie, and M.D. Leveritt. 2012. "The Effects of Different Doses of Caffeine on Endurance Cycling Time Trial Performance." *Journal of Sports Sciences* 30, no. 2, pp. 115–20. doi:10.1080/02640414.2011.632431

Devries, M.C., and S.M. Phillips. 2014. "Creatine Supplementation During Resistance Training in Older Adults-a Meta-Analysis." *Medicine and Science in Sports and Exercise* 46, no. 6, pp. 1194–203. doi:10.1249/MSS.0000000000000220

Dietz, P., R. Ulrich, A. Niess, R. Best, P. Simon, and H. Striegel. 2014. "Prediction Profiles for Nutritional Supplement Use Among Young German elite Athletes." *International Journal of Sport Nutrition and Exercise Metabolism* 24, no. 6, pp. 623–31. doi:10.1123/ijsnem.2014-0009

Erdman, K.A., T.S. Fung, P.K. Doyle-Baker, M.J. Verhoef, and R.A. Reimer. 2007. "Dietary Supplementation of High-Performance Canadian Athletes by Age and Gender." *Clinical Journal of Sport Medicine* 17, no. 6, pp. 458–64. doi:10.1097/JSM.0b013e31815aed33

Geyer, H., M.K. Parr, U. Mareck, U. Reinhart, Y. Schrader, and W. Schanzer. 2004. "Analysis of Non-Hormonal Nutritional Supplements for Anabolic-Androgenic Steroids - Results of an International Study." *International Journal of Sports Medicine* 25, no. 2, pp. 124–29. doi:10.1055/s-2004-819955

Giannopoulou, I., K. Noutsos, N. Apostolidis, I. Bayios, and G.P. Nassis. 2013. "Performance Level Affects the Dietary Supplement Intake of Both Individual and Team Sports Athletes." *Journal of Sports Scienceand Medicine* 12, no. 1, pp. 190–96.

Graham, T.E., E. Hibbert, and P. Sathasivam. 1998. "Metabolic and Exercise Endurance Effects of Coffee and Caffeine Ingestion." *Journal of Applied Physiology (1985)* 85, no. 3, pp. 883–89.

Hodgson, A.B., R.K. Randell, and A.E. Jeukendrup. 2013. "The Metabolic and Performance Effects of Caffeine Compared to Coffee During Endurance Exercise." *PLoS One* 8, no. 4:e59561. doi:10.1371/journal.pone.0059561

Irwin, C., B. Desbrow, A. Ellis, B. O'Keeffe, G. Grant, and M. Leveritt. 2011. "Caffeine Withdrawal and High-Intensity Endurance Cycling Performance." *Journal of Sports Sciences* 29, no. 5, pp. 509–15. doi:10.1080/02640414.2010.541480

Mihic, S., J.R. MacDonald, S. McKenzie, and M.A. Tarnopolsky. 2000. "Acute Creatine Loading Increases Fat-Free Mass, But Does Not Affect Blood Pressure, Plasma Creatinine, or CK Activity in Men and Women." *Medicine and Science in Sports and Exercise* 32, no. 2, pp. 291–96.

Nikolaidis, M.G., C.M. Kerksick, M. Lamprecht, and S.R. McAnulty. 2012. "Does Vitamin C and E Supplementation Impair the Favorable Adaptations of Regular Exercise?" *OxidativeMedicine and Cellular Longevity* 2012:707941. doi:10.1155/2012/707941

Peart, D.J., J.C. Siegler, and R.V. Vince. 2012. "Practical Recommendations for Coaches and Athletes: AMeta-Analysis of Sodium Bicarbonate Use for Athletic Performance." *Journal of Strength and Conditioning Research* 26, no. 7, pp. 1975–83. doi:10.1519/JSC.0b013e3182576f3d

Phillips, S.M., L. Breen, M. Watford, L.M. Burke, S.J. Stear, and L.M. Castell. 2012. "A to Z of Nutritional Supplements: Dietary Supplements, Sports Nutrition Foods and Ergogenic Aids for Health and Performance: Part 32." *British Journal of Sports Medicine* 46, no. 6, pp. 454–56. doi:10.1136/bjsports-2012-091100

Salgado, J.V., P.C. Lollo, J. Amaya-Farfan, and M.P. Chacon-Mikahil. 2014. "Dietary Supplement Usage and Motivation in Brazilian Road Runners." *Journal of International Society of Sports Nutrition* 11, p. 41. doi:10.1186/s12970-014-0041-z

Skaug, A., O. Sveen, and T. Raastad. 2013. "An Antioxidant and Multivitamin Supplement Reduced Improvements in VO2 max." *The Journal of Sports Medicine and Physical Fitness* 54, no. 1, pp. 63–69.

Tarnopolsky, M.A. 2010. "Caffeine and Creatine Use in Sport."*Annals of Nutritionand Metabolism* 57, Suppl 2, pp. 1–8. doi:10.1159/000322696

Torpy, J.M., and E.H. Livingston. 2013. "JAMA Patient Page. Energy Drinks." *JAMA* 309, no. 3, p. 297. doi:10.1001/jama.2012.170614

U.S. Government Accountability Office, ed. 2010. *Herbal Dietary Supplements: Examples of Deceptive or Questionable Marketing Practices and Potential Dangerous Advice*. Washington, DC: U.S. Government Accountability Office.

CHAPTER 8

Common Nutrition Concerns Among Athletes

Rarely does a sports nutrition professional work with an athlete with no special circumstances, and seldom are dietary recommendations as straightforward as those outlined in Chapter 4. Usually the sports nutritionist will need to make adjustments or modifications. This chapter highlights common and important considerations in working with athletes. Many athletes have goals of altering body weight (mass) or body composition, and this requires an individualized and intentional approach so as to maintain health and support optimal performance. The sports nutrition professional must understand the concept of energy balance and why this idea is not so straightforward in implementation. There are considerable concerns regarding weight loss and weight gain practices and so one must be familiar with practical recommendations for safely addressing these goals.

The topic of disordered eating and eating disorders will be addressed, how pathogenic dieting behaviors can result in deleterious effects on health and performance. In fact, athletes are at greater risk for unhealthy nutrition behaviors, especially athletes in weight-sensitive sports. It is important to be able to identify signs and symptoms of these behaviors and refer these athletes to appropriate resources if necessary. Energy availability (EA) is the energy available to the body for physiological processes once the energy expenditure of exercise is accounted for. Athletes in weight-sensitive sports are at greater risk for low EA, which compromises health as well as athletic performance. The sports nutrition professional must have an understanding of these concepts and how to treat athletes with low EA.

Finally, while a balanced, varied, and adequate diet can provide almost all athletes with the micro- and macronutrients needed for performance, there are some athletes at risk for inadequate consumption of specific nutrients. Certain athletes risk inadequate intake of nutrients that are essential for bone health and red blood cell formation, for example, and the sports nutrition professional needs to know how to identify and address these concerns. Overall, vegetarian athletes have been seen to consume nutritionally robust diets, though this balance requires careful planning and intentional intake of targeted nutrients.

Weight Management Goals

Many athletes come to a sports nutrition practitioner with goals related to weight management and body composition. Depending on the sport as well as the individual's current body weight and composition, these goals will vary. Some athletes wish to increase lean body mass (LBM) (muscle) as well as overall body weight, others wish to decrease fat mass (FM) while maintaining LBM, and still other athletes think they can have the best of both worlds and wish to increase muscle mass while simultaneously losing FM and body weight. It is fundamental to understand the specific goals of the athlete, as well as the feasibility of these goals, in order to provide the most effective recommendations.

It is also essential to know *why* athletes are seeking body mass or composition changes. Some individuals are looking to improve overall health, such as an overweight or obese individual who wants to lose weight in order to decrease health risks associated with overweight status. Other athletes want to lose or gain weight because they feel sociocultural pressures to achieve an "ideal" body type. Athletes in weight-sensitive sports, including gravitational sports, aesthetic sports, and weight-class sports, face certain performance pressures and expectations that can drive weight-related goals. This will be discussed in more detail in the following section on "disordered eating and eating disorders among athletes." Some athletes may have unrealistic expectations about how altering body composition will affect their performance; therefore, knowing why an athlete is seeking assistance on weight management is essential for appropriate guidance.

Energy Balance

Recall the principles from Chapter 2 on energy balance. If energy intake equals energy expenditure, weight stays the same. If energy intake is greater than expenditure, weight increases, and if energy intake is lower than expenditure, weight decreases. Because 3,500 kcal equal one pound of body weight, a calorie deficit of 3,500 kcal should result in a weight loss of one pound, and vice versa for weight gain. However, the body does not seem to cooperate with this neat mathematical concept. Swinburn and Ravussin (1993) illustrate this complexity with a classic example (Swinburn and Ravussin 1993). If a 165-lb man consumed an extra 100 kcal every day over a 40-year period, he would theoretically gain 417 lbs! In actuality, he gains 6 lbs over this time frame. What was not accounted for in the theoretical calculation was the increase in energy expenditure resulting from increased body mass. As this man increases in weight from the extra calorie intake, his energy expenditure increases as well. He eventually reaches a point where the calorie surplus equals what his body expends, and thus his weight gain plateaus. If this individual wanted to gain additional weight, he would need to increase his caloric intake even more.

There are many factors influencing the components of energy balance (Manore 2013). Energy balance is affected by total caloric consumption, the macronutrient composition of the diet, amount and type of fiber consumed, timing of food consumption related to exercise, current weight and body composition, and hormonal factors. Energy expenditure is impacted by resting metabolic rate, activities of daily living, exercise, body composition, total calorie content and macronutrient composition of calories, genetics, and overall energy status (such as severe energy restriction). Obviously, it is not just a matter or calories in, calories out.

In addition to the complexity of energy balance, there are other challenges in addressing weight management goals with athletes. To lose or gain weight, energy needs, or energy balance, must be assessed, and then the balance can be tipped in favor of loss or gain. An athlete who wants to lose weight must first know their energy needs to maintain their weight so that calories can be subtracted to create a deficit, for example. Yet, as we saw in Chapter 2, actually measuring an individual's energy expenditure is difficult and various methods have their limitations. This presents a challenge to assessing energy recommendations for weight management.

Athletes in particular have unique challenges for weight loss. Nutrition recommendations for these individuals must supply adequate calories and nutrients to meet the energy and nutrient demands of the sport so as not to compromise performance, let alone health, yet support effective weight loss. While many individuals wanting to lose weight can adjust both the input (food and beverage) and the output (energy expenditure particularly through exercise) sides of the equation, the training demands and training schedule of the athlete may limit what can be modified regarding energy expenditure, thus limiting the range of interventions available. Additionally, weight loss practices should include safe behaviors that do not result in the individual engaging in pathological dieting behaviors or ultimately lead to the development of diagnosed eating disorders.

An Athlete's Approach to Weight Loss

First and foremost, athletes should have realistic expectations about appropriate weight loss. The body composition of the athlete should first be assessed, ideally with a dual energy X-ray absorptiometry (DXA) scan or with skinfold measurements to allow site-specific measurements to be taken and not just an overall body measurement; this can help to better gauge meaningful changes in body composition (Sundgot-Borgen et al. 2013). At the very least, the most accurate assessment that is available to the athlete should be taken (see Chapter 5 on body composition assessment) to establish realistic weight loss goals. Information on genetics and general frame size can further guide what degree of weight loss would be reasonable for an athlete to achieve. In general, it is recommended that males should not go below 5 percent body fat, and females not below 12 percent (Sundgot-Borgen et al. 2013) to maintain overall health and menstrual functioning in women. There are cases where athletes can sustain lower body fat percentages while maintaining overall health, but this needs to be determined on an individual basis.

Athletes should be advised to avoid extreme weight loss practices to avoid detrimental effects to performance and health (Sundgot-Borgen and Garthe 2011). Fad diets and other severely restrictive intakes can compromise an individual's ability to train at high intensities or long duration due to poor glycogen availability, as well as increase the risk of injury due to fatigue and loss of lean tissue. Some weight loss methods can increase the risk of dehydration, especially if the diet is *ketogenic*. Generally, most diets that are intended to reduce body weight in a short period of time also come with risks of overall poor nutrient intake. Following fad diets and weight cycling can also increase the risk of developing disordered eating or eating disorders, as well as increased emotional distress associated with chronic hunger and fatigue.

For a healthful weight loss approach that supports performance, athletes should aim for ~0.5–1 lb (0.25–0.5 kg) of weight loss a week. This can be achieved by a 250–500 caloric deficit a day, either with dietary intake, energy expenditure, or both, depending upon the training status of the athlete. With this approach, athletes can typically meet their nutrient needs (both micro- and macronutrients) while minimizing negative side effects. Ideally, weight loss goals are achieved in the off-season, as this is the best time to address body composition changes. Once an athlete is in competition season, losing weight becomes more difficult because adequate energy is required for peak performance.

Recommendations for Weight Loss in Athletes

The following practices have been shown to support effective and safe weight loss, though these guidelines need to be individualized on a case-by-case basis.

Macronutrient distribution. Even if an athlete wishes to lose weight, they still need to meet basic needs for carbohydrate, protein, and fat to sustain health and immune function as well as support positive training adaptations. Carbohydrate intake should be at least 3 to 5 g/kg/day to meet minimum requirements for maintenance of blood glucose levels and central nervous system function. Protein needs are actually higher for individuals in a calorie deficit. Protein induces a higher rate of thermogenesis, which actually increases caloric expenditure. Protein is also a strong promoter of satiety and feelings of fullness, which is beneficial to individuals who are eating less than the amount required to maintain current body weight. In fact, individuals who are on an energy-restricted diet with low protein intakes (10 to 15 percent of caloric intake) tend to consume more calories compared with individuals with higher protein intakes. Higher protein consumption also helps to preserve LBM and supports muscle protein synthesis, while potentially aiding in fat loss when in a caloric deficit (Phillips 2014). Current research recommends protein consumption of 1.2 to 1.8 g/kg/day, depending upon the sport type, intensity, and duration and training goals of the athlete. However, when caloric intake is severely restricted, protein intake should be as high as 1.8 to 2.7 g of protein/kg body weight. Dietary fat intake is likely the easiest macronutrient to manipulate. Given the density of this nutrient (9 kcal/g versus 4 kcal/g for protein and carbohydrate), eliminating a small amount of fat can significantly decrease total caloric intake. However, fat intake should not go below 20 percent of calories to ensure intake of essential fatty acids is adequate; very-low-fat diets also tend to decrease the satiety of the diet and can make this approach unsustainable.

Focus on a nutrient-dense, low-energy-dense diet. The overall diet should include foods that are high in nutrients, including vitamins and minerals, while avoiding an excess intake of high-energy foods. This can be achieved by inclusion of high fiber, high water content foods that are generally lower in fat. Fruits, vegetables, whole grains, lean proteins including low-fat and nonfat dairy, and focusing on healthy sources of fats will comprise the foundation of this dietary approach. High fiber, high water content foods will help add bulk to the diet and increase satiety while limiting the calorie content. These principles are illustrated by the concept of Volumetrics as proposed by Barbara Rolls (Rolls, Drewnowski, and Ledikwe 2005). The idea here is to keep the volume of food the same while decreasing the calorie content. In fact, this approach has been shown to be an effective method for weight loss while maintaining satisfaction with food, more so than just decreasing portion sizes.

Eating breakfast. Eating breakfast has many benefits to the athlete. Breakfast consumption is a great opportunity to replenish glycogen stores after an overnight fast to ensure carbohydrate availability for exercise. Breakfast is also a time to support increased protein intake, especially since protein consumption should be distributed throughout the day versus one or two large servings. In addition to providing complex carbohydrates and protein, breakfast foods can also be a vital source for important vitamins and minerals, the intakes of which can be compromised on energy-restricted diets. The National Weight Control Registry, which examines behaviors associated with long-term weight loss and maintenance, has found that eating breakfast is a common behavior among individuals with successful weight loss. Breakfast consumption that includes protein can help support appropriate hunger and fullness levels throughout the day and may prevent overeating in the second half of the day.

Timing of Intake. Appropriately timing food intake throughout the day can help successful weight loss. Consuming frequent, small-to-moderate meals throughout the day can help manage hunger and fullness levels while meeting the energy needs of the athlete. This can look like three meals with two to three small snacks, or five to six small meals, whichever is preferable to the athlete. Timing should be coordinated with exercise and training so that individuals are consuming a carbohydrate-containing meal or snack one to four hours before exercise, as well as timing a meal or snack to meet the recovery nutrition needs of the athlete to prevent consumption of an extra meal. The timing of intake is crucial to support the training demands, which, in addition to performance benefits, can also assist muscle mass accrual and favorable body composition changes.

Reducing or eliminating any other unnecessary foods and beverages. The concept of discretionary calories has already been introduced, and individuals with weight loss goals should look to any discretionary calories as an ideal way to reduce total caloric intake. This is especially true for alcoholic beverages and any sugar-sweetened beverages. When individuals consume calories from beverages, versus food sources, they tend to be less satisfied and typically do not compensate for these added calories. That is, food consumption does not decrease even when calorie-containing beverages are consumed. Individuals with a moderate-to-high intake of sugar-sweetened beverages may not notice a decrease in calorie intake when the deficit is achieved by eliminating these drinks.

Reviewing the approach to weight loss. Overall, an athlete should have realistic expectations for weight loss. These recommendations should include healthy eating practices that are sustainable over time while meeting the energy and nutrient demands of the athlete. Questions that can be asked of the athlete to determine the appropriateness of a plan include:

- Is this a diet that can be maintained over a long period of time? Fad and crash diets for example are typically not sustainable.
- Will this approach meet my nutrient and energy needs to sustain the level and volume of training that is required? This includes addressing micro- and macronutrient needs. Strategically timing the intake of nutrients is an important component of the plan to meet these needs.
- Does this plan include a variety of foods and is not overly restrictive? A plan where the individuals feel as though they are chronically "dieting" or engaging in restrained intake can result in the development of disordered eating or diagnosed eating disorders.
- Will this plan meet health and immune function needs, as well as reproductive needs in women?

Obviously, weight management needs to be approached in a sensitive manner utilizing safe practices that are individualized to the needs of each athlete. An approach that promotes 0.5–1 lb weight loss a week can minimize risks associated with severe restriction. The sports nutrition professional should work with the athlete to develop a dietary pattern or meal plan that includes a variety of foods.

An Athlete's Approach to Weight Gain

While the majority of athletes seeking sports nutrition expertise on weight management focus on weight loss, decreasing FM, or both, there are many athlete wishing to increase body mass. Unfortunately, there is significantly less research available on effective methods for weight gain (gain in body mass) in athletes compared to weight loss. This section will highlight what is known as well as provide some practical tips when working with these athletes.

When athletes say they want to gain weight, typically they are referring to an increase in LBM, not FM. A surplus of calories alone will achieve weight gain, but to support LBM accrual, excess calories need to be consumed in conjunction with resistance exercise to stimulate protein synthesis; otherwise excess calories will result in increased FM.

Many athletes appreciate the role that strength training plays in increasing LBM and may spend significant time engaging in resistance exercise to achieve their goals; what is often underappreciated is the role of proper nutrition strategies and the benefit that professional nutrition guidance can provide. For practical reasons, as well as having a fear of gaining excess body fat, athletes may not take a balanced approach to weight gain but rather end up consuming a generally poor diet coupled with protein and other dietary supplements. These athletes likely lack knowledge regarding an appropriate dietary intake and may not seek nutritional counseling. One study that compared LBM accrual in athletes receiving nutritional guidance versus those not receiving guidance found that those who worked with sports nutritionists reported this support was an important criteria for their success; athletes not receiving guidance, however, experienced less success with body mass gains and reported practical challenges that could have been addressed with proper direction.

Recommendations for Weight Gain in Athletes

As with weight loss, it is important to determine an appropriate *rate* of weight gain to optimize results. While sedentary individuals have been found to be able to increase LBM at faster rates, it is known that athletes already engaging in strength training can expect to see a slower rate of increase in LBM (American College of Sports Medicine 2009). That is, athletes with a long history of strength training will have a reduced capacity for increasing LBM and strength. Generally increasing calorie intake to 500 kcal/day greater than energy expenditure is an appropriate approach to take, though a recent study that looked at highly trained resistance athletes speculated that an even slower rate of weight gain at a surplus of 200 to 300 calories/day may be optimal to avoid gains in FM (Garthe et al. 2013).

In addition to a caloric surplus, the composition of the dietary pattern is important. A carbohydrate intake corresponding to 5 to 7 g/kg/day, a higher protein intake of 1.4 to 2.0 g/kg/day, and a fat intake estimating 25 to 30 percent fat seems to support energy and health needs while also providing sufficient protein for synthesis of additional muscle mass. The sports nutrition professional should help the athlete come up with a dietary plan that falls within these recommendations. In conjunction with appropriate macronutrient distribution, adequate fluids should also be consumed, especially with a high protein intake, and food should be distributed equitably throughout the day. As to how caloric intake is distributed, consuming up to seven small-to-moderate meals may be better tolerated by the athlete compared to fewer, excessively large meals.

Achieving increases in daily dietary intake can be challenging for some athletes, in these cases helping the athlete understand the concept of energy density is useful. Consuming foods that are energy dense, that is, have a high energy value per gram, will support a higher caloric intake while avoiding excessively large volumes of food. Returning to the concept of Volumetrics, maintaining a similar volume of food can increase the tolerance for a dietary plan that is changing in calorie content. For example, a strength athlete needing to consume 3,500 kcal/day to increase fat-free mass (FFM) would have to consume unmanageable amounts of fruits and vegetables to meet his energy needs. Fruits and vegetables are important and should be integrated into the plan, but so should energy-dense foods such as nuts and seeds (including nut butters), avocado, healthy vegetable oils. These are all sources of healthy fats, and given that fats are more than twice as calorically dense as carbohydrates and proteins, it makes sense that their inclusion is beneficial. Athletes should avoid excessive amounts of fiber since fiber increases feelings of fullness, potentially making it harder to increase food intake. Additionally, low-fat and even full-fat dairy options can be appropriate in moderate amounts given their higher calorie content for the same volume as their nonfat counterparts.

Timing is an important consideration, and timing recommendations included in Chapter 4 should be integrated into the plan. Particular attention should be paid to proper recovery nutrition practices, with inclusion of a carbohydrate source (40 to 50 g) and a high-quality protein source (20 to 25 g) available within 30 minutes to optimize the postexercise anabolic environment. Another meal of proteins and carbohydrates should be consumed 1 to 2 hours after that to promote continued protein synthesis.

It is not just prescribing the amounts of food and the timing of intake, but the sports nutrition expert can play an integral role in mapping out a schedule for the athlete based upon lifestyle variables and other logistics. It can overwhelm athletes to eat larger amounts of food than what they are used to, so developing an effective nutrition strategy can increase the likelihood of successful implementation. Regular follow-ups and support are also integral to the process.

Exercise prescription may be outside of the scope of sports dietitians depending upon other credentials, but coaches and trainers who provide the training regimen for the athlete should be aware that endurance exercise can mitigate some of the benefits received from resistance training in efforts to increase LBM. Individuals whose training plan includes endurance exercise are more likely to show a lower response to the effects of resistance training, so this should be considered by the athlete in setting realistic expectations for LBM gains (American College of Sports Medicine 2009).

There is no guarantee that an increase in body weight will be the result of 100 percent LBM accrual. Effective nutrition counseling can enhance this process, but even athletes who are successful at increasing body weight, through recommended nutritional strategies, still may see part of those increases as a result of additional FM. This is particularly true for elite-level resistance athletes, and this can at least partly be explained by the decreased capacity for LBM accrual in these athletes (Garthe et al. 2013). Nonetheless, safe and healthful strategies for increasing LBM should be promoted and have been shown to be effective.

Disordered Eating and Eating Disorders Among Athletes

Defining Disordered Eating and Eating Disorders

Disordered eating and eating disorders are serious psychological issues that can have severe effects on physiological and mental health. According to the fifth edition of the *Diagnostic and Statistical Manual of Mental Disorders (DSM-5)*, clinical eating disorders are diagnosable psychiatric conditions including: anorexia nervosa, bulimia nervosa, binge eating disorder, and other specified feeding or eating disorders (OSFED). Eating disorders are characterized by disturbance in the way one view's their body, and body weight and shape unduly influence thoughts and behaviors. Individuals with eating disorders have a preoccupation with food and body weight and this results in unhealthy behaviors including starvation, binging, purging, and excessive exercise.

There is a spectrum of eating behaviors that individuals fall along. At one end of the spectrum, there are healthy eating behaviors characterized by appropriate macro- and micronutrient intake as well as being characterized by the concepts of balance, variety, and moderation. Overall, these individuals have a healthy relationship with food. The other end of the eating spectrum would include clinically diagnosed eating disorders. Disordered eating behaviors include pathological eating behaviors that fall along the continuum. Disordered eating behaviors may begin with healthy intentions to lose weight or body fat but somehow these behaviors progress into dangerous behaviors such as restrictive eating, chronic dieting, using forms of purging (diuretics, laxatives, vomiting, diet pills), excessive sweating with sweat suits and saunas, or excessive exercise. Disordered eating may include exhibiting some, but not all, of the criteria and behaviors used in the diagnosis of eating disorders. Nonetheless, disordered eating is a significant risk factor for the development of an eating disorder and without intervention it is possible disordered eating will progress to an eating disorder.

Prevalence and Risk Factors of Disordered Eating and Eating Disorders

Determining actual rates of disordered eating and eating disorders among athletes is challenging for many reasons, including inconsistency in definitions used, different methodologies used to assess prevalence, prevalence variability within different sport types, just to name a few. In general, disordered eating and eating disorders appear to be more common in athletes versus nonathletes, and the higher the level of performance, typically, the greater the prevalence (Bratland-Sanda and Sundgot-Borgen 2013). Women have a higher prevalence compared to men, though it is believed disordered eating and eating disorders are more likely to go undiagnosed in men. According to the criteria set forth by the previous edition of the *DSM (IV)*, the most common eating disorder diagnosis among athletes was eating disorders not otherwise specified; however, this remains to be confirmed by the *DSM-V*. Overall, results from studies that have examined several athletic populations have found a prevalence of all eating disorders that ranges from 18 to 45 percent in female athletes (Nichols et al. 2007; Sundgot-Borgen 1994), and 0 to 28 percent among male athletes (Torstveit and Sundgot-Borgen 2005).

Athletes participating in weight-sensitive sports that emphasize leanness, such as gravitational sports, aesthetic sports, and weight-class sports, have a higher prevalence of disordered eating and eating disorders. Gravitational sport athletes must move their body against gravity and thus performance may be restricted by additional body mass. Athletes who participate in endurance running and cycling, cross-country skiing, and ski jumping often feel pressure to decrease body mass while maintaining a high power-to-weight ratio. In aesthetic sports, physique and physical presentation are part of what is being judged, and thus can increase pressure to maintain a certain body image. These sports include gymnastics, figure skating, and other dancing sports. Weight-class athletes, such as wrestlers, combat sport athletes (judo, boxing, taekwondo) and lightweight rowers, have actual weight requirements for their sport and thus face external demands to achieve a specific weight.

Athletes in these sports may feel pressures from coaches, parents, or just from themselves, to reach performance measures that they believe require body composition and weight modifications. Due to these pressures, athletes in these sports are at higher risk for development of disordered eating and eating disorders. Other risk factors include personality factors such as perfectionism and (over-)compliance, early start of sport-specific training, injuries and traumatic events, and coaching behavior that includes preoccupation with body weight. Of course, there are other cultural, individual, family and genetic or biochemical factors that can increase one's risk (Sundgot-Borgen et al. 2013). While it is outside of the scope of this text to examine each risk factor individually, it is important to understand the development of disordered eating and eating disorders is quite multifactorial.

Impact of Disordered Eating and Eating Disorders on Performance

Given the fact that in weight-sensitive sports up to 94 percent of elite athletes report dieting and use of extreme weight-controlling measures prior to competition, it is essential to understand the performance effects of these behaviors (Sundgot-Borgen and Garthe 2011). In general, the type, frequency, severity, and duration of behaviors used to lose weight will determine the physiological and psychological effects, as will an individual's overall health status, weight, and body composition prior to weight loss (Sundgot-Borgen et al. 2013).

Individuals who severely restrict their intake or use fasting methods for weight loss are likely to experience poor performance outcomes related to inadequate energy and nutrient intake. These individuals are likely to exhibit overall weakness, decreased force production, inability to cope with sport pressures, and increased risk for injury and illness. Long-term low EA may also result in a decrease in maximum oxygen consumption, negatively impacting aerobic capacity. Restrictive intakes may also result poor performance due to nutrient deficiencies, as seen with iron deficiency anemia (IDA) (to be discussed later in this chapter).

Individuals taking laxatives, enemas, or diuretics are at risk for dehydration, electrolyte imbalances, and constipation specifically with laxative use; this may affect performance by impairing mental acuity and other dehydration-related effects. Additionally, diuretics are classified as doping and can exclude athletes from competition. Athletes engaging in self-induced vomiting may also experience negative dehydration-related performance effects, and are especially prone to electrolyte abnormalities. Excessive exercise can result in poor recovery and these athletes may experience prolonged fatigue, increased risk for illnesses, and overuse injuries. Overall, severe dieting behaviors can significantly impair performance and need to be addressed.

Addressing Disordered Eating and Eating Disorders

The American College of Sports Medicine (ACSM), the American Academy of Pediatrics (AAP), the International Olympic Committee (IOC), and the National Athletic Trainer Association (NATA) have urged national and international sports federations to develop and implement policies and procedures to address and eliminate unhealthy weight loss practices. Additionally, a research working group under the auspices of the IOC Medical Commission in 2013 published a review and position statement titled "How to minimize the health risks to athletes who compete in weight-sensitive sports review and position statement on behalf of the Ad Hoc Research Working Group on Body Composition, Health and Performance, under the auspices of the IOC Medical Commission" (Sundgot-Borgen et al. 2013). This paper should be referenced for more comprehensive guidelines on addressing the complex issues of working with athletes in weight-sensitive sports. Some key points will be identified here.

Practitioners working with these athletes should be knowledgeable about the growth and development needs of athletes, as well as understand the interactions between nutrition, dieting and EA, and body composition and performance. These practitioners should be able to identify disordered eating and eating disorders, detect signs and symptoms, and refer athletes to appropriate professionals for diagnosis. There are a host of signs and symptoms associated with disordered eating or eating disorders, which include but are not limited to athletes presenting with symptoms of long-term restrictive eating practices including chronic low energy levels and fatigue, recurrent illness or injury or both, menstrual irregularities, or a decrease in performance; or, the athlete presents with more acute symptoms of unhealthy dieting practices that include headaches, dizziness, fatigue, and rapid weight loss. Prompt detection of unhealthy practices is essential, because early identification and treatment is crucial for improved outcomes and recovery for the athlete.

These individuals should work in a team environment for optimal treatment outcomes. This includes a medical professional to manage any medical complications, a registered dietitian (ideally sports dietitian) who can establish healthy eating patterns and help the athlete to develop a healthier relationship with food, a therapist to help address psychological distress and help identify underlying causes of the eating disorder, and potentially an athletic trainer, dentist, or other health professionals, depending upon the extent of the disorder and its manifestations.

Sports nutrition experts should be well versed in practices that support healthy weight loss, including those outlined in the previous section on weight management. Particularly with weight-sensitive sports, these athletes should have their body composition assessed at the beginning of the season and should be monitored on a regular basis. Female athletes need at least 30 to 45 kcal/kg of FFM to ensure adequate EA. This will be further discussed in the section on the female athlete triad, concepts with which these practitioners should be quite familiar.

Assessment of athletes at risk should include the ABCDE assessment (Sundgot-Borgen et al. 2013). A represents anthropometric information (height, weight, body composition, etc.) that should be collected, B refers to relevant biochemical data (such as a complete blood count (CBC), complete metabolic panel, iron profile, urine analysis, etc.), C includes clinical information (history, medications, physical examination), D stands for dietary data (quality, quantity, timing), as well as collecting Environmental (E) information (energy expenditure, training plan, environmental factors, etc.). A more detailed description is available in the Institute of Medicine (IOM) position paper. In this paper, there is also included information on criteria for raising alarm as well as "no start" decisions (Sundgot-Borgen et al. 2013). This provides objective measures that health professionals can use to assess if an athlete needs to stop sport participation until they are at a more stable place that will not compromise their health.

In summary, sport nutrition professionals should be aware of the health risks and performance effects of extreme dieting behaviors and diagnosed eating disorders. These practitioners should be able to help athletes achieve body composition and weight goals in a healthy manner, as well as be aware of signs and symptoms of when healthy behaviors evolve into pathogenic behaviors. If the sports nutrition practitioner is not confident in their ability to work with these athletes then they should have resources available for appropriate referrals.

The Female Athlete Triad and Relative Energy Deficiency in Sport

Components of the Triad

The term "female athlete triad" (or, the "Triad") was first coined in 1992, and since that time diagnosis of this medical condition has evolved into a complex interaction of different indexes of health. The three components that comprise the Triad are (1) low EA with or without disordered eating; (2) menstrual dysfunction; and (3) low bone mineral density (BMD). It is now understood that low EA underpins the other two components. Thus, it is essential to have an understanding of EA. The Triad is most commonly seen in athletes who participate in the weight-sensitive sports outlined earlier, probably as a result of the relative importance of leanness in these sports.

Energy Availability: The Underlying Cause

EA is the amount of dietary energy remaining after exercise training for all other physiological functions each day (De Souza et al. 2014). EA = Energy Intake (EI) in kcal minus the energy cost of exercise (kcal) relative to FFM in kg. Simplified, EA (kcal/kg FFM/day) = [EI (kcal/day) – exercise EE (kcal/day)]/kg FFM. A total of 45 kcal/kg FFM/day is considered to be sufficient for meeting the physiological needs of the body once the energy demands of training have been accounted for. Low EA is considered to be 30 kcal/kg FFM/day or less, as this is the threshold below which harmful changes occur in reproductive, metabolic, and bone health. Disordered eating and eating disorders are not always the cause of low EA, since inadequate EI may merely be due to a lack of understanding by the athlete as to their actual energy needs. However, it is more commonly the case that there are disordered eating practices underlying low EA.

In between 30 and 45 kcal/kg FFM/day represents suboptimal intake that may result in hormonal, metabolic, and functional perturbations, though in this range there are less likely to be clinical manifestations. It should be noted that these values are not clear-cut; different physiological functions (hormonal responses and markers of bone formation) will respond differently at different EA levels, and there will be interindividual variations in response to low EA. Thus, values of 45 kcal/kg FFM/day and 30 kcal/kg FFM/day should be viewed as estimates to approximate EA adequacy.

Low EA is thought to contribute to the Triad, particularly menstrual and bone health. Low EA plays a causal role in menstrual disturbances. Whereas adequate EA supports *eumenorrhea*, low EA may result in menstrual disturbances such as luteal phase defects and anovulation, as well as *oligomenorrhea, primary amenorrhea,* or *secondary amenorrhea.* Essentially, low EA disrupts an important hormonal cascade of the hypothalamus that alters menstrual functioning. This is known as functional hypothalamus amenorrhea. For a clinician to ascertain if low EA is at the root of menstrual dysfunction, other potential etiologies need to be ruled out.

Low EA by itself, and through its causal role in low estrogen levels (hypoestrogenism), has negative musculoskeletal effects through its disruption of bone remodeling. This can result in bone stress injuries, including stress fractures, and ultimately can increase the risk for low BMD. Unfortunately, depending upon the extent of damage, these effects may be irreversible.

A recent effort has been made to shift from using the term Female Athlete Triad, to using "Relative Energy Deficiency in Sport" (RED-S). Relative energy deficiency connotes that low EA can occur even when there is no energy deficit; that is, EI and total energy expenditure are "balanced" (Mountjoy et al. 2014). RED-S proponents believe that use of the term Triad results in a more limited view of low EA, and instead of just a triad of three entities, this clinical phenomenon is a medical syndrome affecting many aspects of functioning. There is also concern that the Triad fails to capture the negative effects of energy deficiency in males, and that using the term "Athlete" in the Female Athlete Triad may restrict other active individuals from being included. It has yet to be seen if RED-S will replace the Triad terminology, though there are some concepts that should be considered.

There are indeed other effects of low EA than just the impact on bone and menstrual health (and the Triad proponents agree with this), including detriments to metabolic health, immunity, protein synthesis, cardiovascular and psychological health (Mountjoy et al. 2014), all which need to be addressed in athletes exhibiting low EA. Additionally, while there is a paucity of research, there is some support for low EA in male athletes and evidence that it impairs endocrine and bone health. However, as of yet, research has not delineated the cut-off values for low EA in men due to lack of sufficient evidence. Thus, given the potential consequences it has on overall health, sports nutrition experts need to be able to identify and treat both males and females with low EA.

Practitioners should also be familiar with and able to identify athletes at risk for muscle dysmorphia. Muscle dysmorphia is a specific type of body dysmorphia most commonly seen among male athletes and is characterized by a fear of being too small; these individuals often perceive themselves to be smaller than they actually are. There is often a hypervigilance to even small deviations from their perceived ideal (typically a large, muscular figure), and they may ignore feedback that their body image is not consistent with reality. While it is outside of the scope of this text to go into further treatment recommendations, these individuals should be referred to a mental health professional as would anyone dealing with diagnosed eating disorders. Because of their drive to increase muscle mass at all costs, these individuals are at greater risk for substance use and excessive exercise. This needs to be addressed to avoid potential negative effects to their health.

Treatment of Low EA and Related Health Indexes

Depending upon the medical and nutritional status of the athlete, participation in sport may be discontinued until the individual is at a more medically and nutritionally stable place. Table 8.1 provides an assessment that can be used to determine if continued participation in sport is recommended, keeping in mind the health of the athlete must be the number one priority. Regardless of participation status, addressing and correcting EA is the cornerstone of treatment for these athletes.

Treatment of low EA needs to include an increase in EI, a decrease in energy expenditure, or both. The goal is to get an athlete's EA to at least 45 kcal/kg of FFM per day, keeping in mind this value pertains to calories needed in addition to those expended during physical activity. If FFM can be determined, the athlete's energy needs can be calculated and estimated. However, since there are limitations to accurately assessing EA in athletes, a more practical recommendation for increasing EA is to increase caloric intake by 300 to 600 kcals/day and to decrease energy expenditure as appropriate (Mountjoy et al. 2014).

Once EA is sufficient (a process that my take several months or more), menstrual function typically normalizes since weight regain is one of the

Table 8.1 *"No Start" Criteria: should athletes be allowed to participate in sport as developed by the Norwegian Olympic Training Center*

Alarm criteria	Observations
Women: BMI <18.5 or body fat % <12% and primary or secondary amenorrhea Men: BMI <18.5 or body fat % <5% and low testosterone	*BMI measures relative body weight but does not accurately assess body composition; % body fat is based upon DXA yet there lacks accurate field measurements*
Amenorrhea ≥ 6 months (>3 months for athletes <18 years)	*Amenorrhea as caused by low EA; athletes using oral contraceptives with regular cycles and < 12% body fat should be considered to meet "alarm criteria"*
Reduced BMD, Z-score ≤ −1	*BMD values from L2 to L4*
Athletes with physical complications based upon medical assessment	*Includes electrolyte imbalances, stress fractures, and fatigue*
Uncooperative athletes or those showing a lack of progress	
Athletes having a negative effect on other team members such as unhealthy dieting behaviors and unstable mood	*Includes behaviors such as binging, purging, restrictive eating, excessive focus on food and weight*
Athletes unable to maintain positive energy balance over time, lack of responsiveness to training, or consistent fatigue and intolerance	
No start criteria	
Athletes meeting diagnostic criteria for diagnosed eating disorder (Anorexia Nervosa, Bulimia Nervosa, OSFED) and electrolyte disturbances	
Athletes with severe physical complications associated with weight loss and lack of EA	*Includes cardiac dysrhythmias, major edema, fainting*
At least 3 of the "alarm criteria" outlined previously	

Source: Adapted from The Malnourished athlete—guidelines for interventions (Skarderud et al. 2012).

greatest predictors of normal menstrual functioning. Adequate EI in of itself, as well as its effects on normalizing estrogen levels, can improve BMD, though not all losses may be recovered. Resistance training should be included as a treatment for improving BMD, given its role as a stimulus for increasing bone density, as well as recommendations for appropriate vitamin supplementation. Bone nutrient supplementation is outlined in the following section.

For individuals with eating disorders, simply adding calories to the diet may not be successful given the psychological distress associated with eating. The practitioner(s) need to ascertain the scope of disordered eating or eating disorder that may exist and utilize the treatment team approach as outlined in the earlier section. The role of the dietitian or nutritionist in this process includes the principles outlined for dietary management of disordered eating and eating disorders. The nutritionist should help to ensure appropriate macro- and micronutrient intake as well as adequate EI; they also serve a role in normalizing food behaviors. Progress may be slow and can take months, even years if the eating disorder is severe. The athlete should be educated on the importance of proper nutrition intake for overall health, for proper bone and menstrual functioning, as well as the role nutrition plays on performance. The nutritionist can support the development of a healthy relationship with food, including the integration of principles of mindful eating and intuitive eating. Finding what motivates the athlete to work toward adequate EA will be useful in establishing goals and objectives.

Overall low EA is the underlying factor in the Female Athlete Triad and RED-S. Health consequences of low EA are significant and a team approach is needed to address the various physiological disturbances. The sports nutritionist plays an integral role in supporting the athlete in achieving sufficient EA, both through dietary recommendations and meal planning, as well as by normalizing healthy eating patterns. The process is ongoing and can take an extended period of time, but it is essential the athlete understands the significant role nutrition plays in optimizing health and performance.

Nutrient Needs and Deficiencies

Nutrient Needs of Athletes

The Dietary Reference Intakes (DRI) developed by the IOM establish nutrient recommendations for the U.S. population, and this includes recommended vitamin and mineral intakes. The Recommended Dietary

Allowance (RDA) is the dietary intake level adequate for 98 percent of the healthy U.S. population, and when there is insufficient research an Adequate Intake (AI) is established until more research is available. The Tolerable Upper Intake Level (UL) is the maximum amount of a nutrient that can be consumed without any adverse effects.

There is a question as to whether or not the recommended micronutrient intakes established by the DRIs are sufficient to meet the needs of athletes. There is some argument that athletes have increased needs, at least for some nutrients, given the increased demands placed upon their bodies as a result of training and competition. In general, if an athlete consumes a balanced and varied diet as proposed by Chapter 6 and meets the increased energy needs, then in most cases, athletes will consume an appropriate amount of vitamins and minerals to meet their needs. This emphasizes the importance in educating athletes on focusing on nutrient-dense food choices.

Meeting individual nutrient needs also illustrates the importance of sufficient calories and individual macronutrients. Indeed, athletes with a restrictive intake that do not meet their energy needs are also at greater risk for an inadequate consumption of macronutrients and micronutrients. In a review that examined the nutrient intake of athletes, it was found that individuals with a low energy consumption were more likely to have an inadequate intake of calcium, iron, magnesium, zinc, and vitamin B12 (Economos, Bortz, and Nelson 1993); this finding has been corroborated by other research as well (Beals 2002; Gropper, Sorrels, and Blessing 2003).

While the questionable benefits of supplement use was addressed in Chapter 7, it is appropriate to reiterate that if an athlete's diet is characterized by nutrient-dense food choices and include sufficient energy, then the athlete is likely to be consuming sufficient vitamins and minerals. In this case, a multivitamin or other nutrient supplement would not be warranted. If, however, the athlete is on an energy-restricted diet, thereby making it harder to meet their nutrient needs, consuming a multivitamin would be judicial for ensuring AI, as long as it does not exceed DRI values.

The purpose of the following information is to highlight nutrients of concern for athletes and to provide relevant recommendations. Specific attention will be paid to nutrients essential for bone health, given the demands that sports may place on the musculoskeletal system; and iron status in athletes, due to the higher prevalence of iron deficiency among athletes.

Nutrients Needed for Bone Health

Bone is a dynamic and an active organ that requires adequate energy and nutrients for optimal health. Bone is an organic matrix—half of which is composed of protein—that holds various minerals, particularly calcium and phosphate. This matrix makes bone dense so that it can support the weight of the body and protect internal organs. Bone is constantly turning over, with old bone resorbed through the action of cells called osteoclasts, and new bone being laid down by cells known as osteoblasts. If the rate of bone deposition is greater than bone resorption, BMD increases, and if bone resorption outpaces bone deposition then BMD will decrease. While many factors will impact an individual's BMD, including genetics, hormonal factors, and environmental factors, nutrition plays a significant role modulating bone turnover.

Individuals should be encouraged to view dietary habits as a way of optimizing their bone health, since nutrition is one variable an athlete has control over, whereas other factors (especially genetics) cannot be changed. Micronutrients important for bone health include calcium, vitamin D, vitamin K, Vitamin A, magnesium, phosphorous, fluoride, iron, zinc; protein and fat (especially omega-3 fatty acids) are essential macronutrients. Further, sufficient energy consumption is required for positive bone turnover. Bones have a sensor that detects energy status, and when caloric intake is insufficient, there is increased bone resorption and decreased bone formation. Protein's metabolites, amino acids, help stimulate bone formation; omega-3 fatty acids help moderate inflammation that can be detrimental to bone formation. Protein and fat needs have been addressed in Chapter 4 and will not be discussed here. This section focuses on calcium and vitamin D since calcium intake is most likely to be inadequate among athletes, and vitamin D status is commonly insufficient or deficient.

Calcium. Calcium is an important mineral deposited in the bone matrix helping to give bone its strength. The RDA for calcium is shown

Table 8.2 RDA for calcium and vitamin D

Age or life stage	Calcium		Vitamin D	
	RDA	UL	RDA	UL
9–13 years old	1,300	3,000	600	4,000
14–18 years old	1,300	3,000	600	4,000
19–30 years old	1,000	2,500	600	4,000
31–50 years old	1,000	2,500	600	4,000
51–70 year old males	1,000	2,000	600	4,000
51–70 year old females	1,200	2,000	600	4,000
> 70 years old	1,200	2,000	800	4,000
14–18, pregnant or lactating	1,300	3,000	600	4,000
19–50, pregnant or lactating	1,000	2,500	600	4,000

in Table 8.2, which depicts how calcium needs are higher in adolescence and later in life, with a slight dip in the mid-years. The increased amounts represent periods of increased needs related to physiological processes of the lifecycle. During adolescence, needs are increased due to the rapid rate of bone deposition, particularly surrounding *menarche*. In fact, during this period, bone is deposited at a rate four times higher than the rate of deposition in other stages of life. Thus meeting increased calcium needs during this time is crucial for reaching peak bone mass, and those who fail to meet their calcium needs are at much greater risk of not achieving peak bone mass. This can significantly increase their likelihood of developing osteoporosis and an increased fracture risk later in life (Rizzoli 2014).

Calcium needs decrease slightly until women reach menopause, though this is not to suggest calcium intake is not as important during this "mid-life" period. In fact, adequate calcium intake between adolescence and menopause helps to maintain the bone mass that has been achieved and attenuate the rate of bone loss. Finally, during menopause, estrogen levels decrease, resulting in an increased rate of bone loss, and an increased rate of bone turnover. This increases the need for calcium at this stage.

As described earlier, athletes are often seen to have inadequate intakes of calcium, especially adolescent athletes for whom adequate intake is so crucial. These athletes should be educated on calcium-rich foods and

Table 8.3 Calcium content in certain foods

Food or beverage source	Serving size	Calcium (mg)
Milk (skim, low fat, whole)	1 cup	300
Cottage cheese	0.5 cup	65
Yogurt	1 cup	450
String cheese	1 stick	200
Ice cream	0.5 cup	100
Spinach, cooked	0.5 cup	120
Kale, raw	1 cup	55
Broccoli, cooked	0.5 cup	90
Figs, dried	0.5 cup	150
Orange juice, fortified	1 cup	300
Soymilk, fortified	1 cup	200–400
White beans, cooked	0.5 cup	70
Tofu, regular	0.5 cup/4 oz	120–390
Fortified cereals	0.5–1 cup	250–1,000
Almonds	1 oz	80
Canned salmon with bones	3 oz	170–210
Blackstrap molasses	1 tablespoon	135

given practical suggestions for integrating these foods into their diets. Table 8.3 shows the calcium content of various foods. Dairy foods in general are a great source of calcium with a high bioavailability and can be a great way to increase calcium intake; for athletes with lactose intolerance or who choose to abstain from dairy foods, dairy alternatives are typically fortified with calcium and can contribute to overall intake.

If, upon reviewing a food log it is apparent an individual has a low calcium intake through food sources and is not able to increase their intake of these foods, calcium supplements should be recommended. These athletes may not need the full recommended calcium intake to come from supplements; rather, the nutritionist first can assess how much they get on a daily basis (on average) and can then supplement that which is not being consumed. For example, a 14-year-old female soccer player chooses not to eat dairy but drinks two glasses of soy milk (fortified with calcium) a day and has a moderate intake of green leafy vegetables. Her estimated intake of calcium is roughly 700 mg/day. Thus, she would only need one 600 mg calcium supplement to meet her recommended intake of 1,300 mg/day. This highlights the importance of the dietary assessment in order to ascertain appropriate nutrient recommendations.

Vitamin D. Vitamin D is one of the more debated nutrients in regard to its impact on many physiological processes, including health and performance parameters relevant to athletes. Vitamin D is often known as the "sun vitamin" because we get most of our vitamin D from sun exposure. Small amounts are found in food sources (see Table 8.4), though the amount in these foods is variable and most individuals do not consume adequate quantities of these foods to meet their daily needs. Even the amount that we get from the sun varies, depending upon geographical location, latitude, seasonality, skin color, age, use of sunscreen, and other variables. Given the dearth of dietary sources, and the variability in optimal sun exposure, there is concern that many individuals, including athletes, are in poor vitamin D status. In fact, it is estimated that up to 77 percent of Americans are considered to be "insufficient" in vitamin D (serum 25(OH)D levels < 32 ng/dL) (Ginde, Liu, and Camargo 2009). Status among athletes depends upon many of the variables listed previously, including geographic location and type of sport, though it is thought that athletes have comparable vitamin D status as the rest of the population. Indoor athletes are considered at greater risk than outdoor athletes due to their lack of sun exposure.

Vitamin D's role in calcium regulation and supporting calcium absorption has been established for some time. It is in reference to this function of vitamin D that the IOM established the RDA (see Table 8.2), and thus

Table 8.4 Food sources of Vitamin D

Food or beverage source	Serving size	Vitamin D (IU)
Salmon (sockeye)	3 oz	447
Canned tuna in water	3 oz	154
Orange juice fortified with Vitamin D	1 cup	137
Milk (skim, low fat, whole), fortified	1 cup	115–124
Egg, whole	1 egg	41
Cod liver oil	1 tablespoon	1,360
Yogurt, fortified with 20% of Daily Value	6 oz	80

the amount of vitamin D needed for other physiological functions may not be captured by the RDA. Some of these other functions of vitamin D pertaining to athletes include its role immune function, protein synthesis, muscle function, inflammatory response, cellular growth, and regulation of skeletal muscle (Ogan and Pritchett 2013). Vitamin D's role in these other processes is still being understood, and as of yet there is insufficient evidence to raise the RDA. There is debate surrounding this, and many individuals believe the IOM's recommendations are only enough to prevent deficiency, but are not enough to achieve optimal vitamin D status.

There is also debate surrounding definitions of vitamin D status. The IOM defines deficiency as serum 25(OH)D less than 20 ng/mL. Many researchers and practitioners believe that insufficiency, however, is a serum 25(OH)D level between 20 and 32 ng/dL, and optimal status is marked by serum 25(OH)D levels of greater than 40 ng/dL. These are not standardized definitions, however, and thus makes it challenging to assess deficiency, insufficiency, and optimal status in athletes. Given that these are the most commonly used definitions, this is what will be used in this text. These ranges also imply that not only would individuals, including athletes, want to prevent deficiency, but would at the very least want to avoid insufficiency if not aim for optimal status. Because there are challenges with meeting vitamin D needs with food sources and sun exposure, there is question as to whether athletes should supplement with vitamin D to support optimal status (or at least avoid insufficiency or deficiency).

A recent review identified a strong relationship between vitamin D and muscle strength, mass, and function (Girgis et al. 2013). There are vitamin D receptors right in skeletal muscle, and research has demonstrated cellular and genomic mechanisms linking vitamin D with muscle function. How this translates to performance is less clear. Most studies have looked at measures of strength, with the results being mixed. Some intervention studies show improvements in strength when supplemented with vitamin D, some do not. These mixed results can partly be explained by issues of methodology and definitions. For example, the vitamin D status of the athlete at the beginning of the intervention seems to impact the outcome. As mentioned, definitions of status (deficiency, insufficiency, and optimal status) are not standardized, which creates problems in trying to compare results of different studies.

Based on the current state of research, there is insufficient evidence to develop a standard supplementation protocol. Athletes, especially indoor athletes, should be encouraged to get their vitamin D status checked, especially during periods when poor status is most likely (in the winter months). Supplementation should be initiated if an athlete is deficient, and there is reason to support supplementation to avoid insufficiency as well (serum 25(OH)D levels > 32 ng/dL). Because toxicity of vitamin D is rare and would only result from excessive supplementation, consuming food sources in vitamin D would be prudent, such as salmon and fatty fish, especially given the benefit of these foods for a variety of reasons previously described.

Iron Status and Athletes

Iron is a micronutrient with many essential functions in the body that are particularly relevant to athletic performance. Perhaps one of its most vital roles pertains to its distribution of oxygen throughout the body as a component of hemoglobin and myoglobin. Iron is a constituent of mitochondrial enzymes required for oxidative phosphorylation, and thus aerobic metabolism relies upon this mineral as well. It is through these mechanisms of oxygen delivery and oxidative capacity that it can be understood how poor iron status can result in feelings of fatigue and ultimately reduce endurance capacity.

Iron deficiency is the most common nutrient deficiency worldwide. In the United States alone, 16 percent of premenopausal women face iron deficiency, and 3 to 5 percent of women have iron deficiency anemia (IDA) (Cogswell et al. 2009). IDA is defined as hemoglobin (Hgb) levels <12 g/dL in women and <13 g/dL in men. Individuals at risk for iron deficiency include menstruating women (due to menstrual blood loss), vegetarians, and individuals at stages of the lifecycle involving growth and development including childhood, adolescence, and pregnancy and lactation. Because exercise can increase iron requirements by up to 70 percent (Whiting and Barabash 2006), athletes and especially female athletes are at much greater risk of iron deficiency. In fact, female athletes are twice as likely to suffer IDA as their nonathletic counterparts. Athletes may exhibit low iron stores for a variety of reasons, including plasma volume expansion, low dietary iron intake, low iron bioavailability, and excessive iron excretion or loss (such as through red blood cell hemolysis, sweat, and hematuria) (Goodman et al. 2011).

Indeed, athletic performance has been shown to suffer in the presence of IDA. Poor oxygen transport as seen with reduced Hgb levels impairs VO_{2max} in athletes, in some studies by up to 50 percent in the presence of IDA. Additionally, with compromised tissue oxidative capacity, endurance performance is reduced. What is less clear is if athletes who are iron deficient in the absence of IDA experience impaired performance. Research is mixed on this topic, in part due to methodological issues as well as inconsistencies of definitions of iron deficiency; this requires further investigation.

The RDA for iron is 8 mg for ages 9 to 13 years; 11 and 15 mg for males and females of ages 14 to 18 years, respectively; and 8 and 18 mg for males and females of ages 19 to 50 years, respectively. Iron can be consumed from meats, as well as from plant sources such as legumes, leafy greens, nuts, and fortified grain products. There are two different dietary sources of iron, heme iron, and nonheme iron. While overall iron bioavailability is low, heme iron found in meat (comprising 40 percent of the iron in meat) is significantly more bioavailable than nonheme iron found in plant foods. This accounts for why vegetarians have a much greater need for iron (see following section on Vegetarian Athletes). See Table 8.5 for dietary sources of iron. Consuming nonheme iron along with Vitamin C (supplemental or food forms), or consumption of meat, poultry, and seafood at the same time can improve nonheme iron absorption. Phytates found in grains and legumes impede iron absorption, as well as calcium, tea, and coffee.

Athletes do not always consume adequate iron from dietary sources, which can be due to dietary preferences, dietary approaches such as vegetarianism, and overall inadequate EI due to restrictive eating patterns or efforts toward weight loss. Recognizing that intake may be suboptimal, athletes have higher iron losses and thus increased iron requirements, and understanding iron's role in achieving optimal athletic performance emphasizes the importance of accurately assessing iron status and helping athletes achieve optimal iron stores. However, this is not always a straightforward process.

Table 8.5 Iron content in certain foods

Food or beverage source	Serving size	Iron (mg)
Breakfast cereals fortified with 100% of the RDA for iron	1 serving (check label)	18
Oysters, cooked	3 oz	8
White beans, cooked	0.5 cup	4
Lentils, cooked	0.5 cup	3
Spinach, cooked	0.5 cup	3
Tofu, firm	4 oz	3
Stewed tomatoes	0.5 cup	2
Baked potato with skin	1 medium	2
Beef, trimmed	3 oz	2
Chicken, roasted	3 oz	1
Whole wheat spaghetti, cooked	1 cup	1
Broccoli, cooked	0.5 cup	1

Hemoglobin (Hgb) levels are used to diagnose IDA, though there is a question as to whether this measure accurately captures deficiency in athletes. This belief is supported by studies showing improvements in oxidative metabolism in athletes supplemented with iron when Hgb levels were low but nonanemic (Schoene et al. 1983). Serum ferritin is a more sensitive measure of iron status and can identify iron *depletion* (when serum ferritin stores are depleted but hemoglobin levels are still in the normal range) and subclinical iron deficiency sooner than Hgb (or hematocrit) can. Serum ferritin levels <12 g/dL define IDA, though many health practitioners believe serum ferritin between 12 and 20 g/dL indicate iron deficiency, and aim for a serum ferritin level of at least 30 ng/dL to ensure adequate iron stores. One limitation of both these measures is that both Hgb and serum ferritin do not actually measure iron stores, but rather measure iron levels in the blood, with the assumption that as stored iron decreases so do levels in the blood. Being able to directly measure iron stores would provide a much better feedback regarding the iron status of athletes.

Iron supplementation. Routine iron supplementation irrespective of iron status is not warranted due to concerns of iron overload. Iron induces oxidative damage and production of free radicals, which can eventually result in organ and cellular damage in individuals consuming high amounts of iron. Iron overload is most common among individuals supplementing with large amounts of iron, and is more frequently seen in men versus women. Thus, individuals in good iron status should not routinely take iron supplements, especially given that for these individuals there is not a performance benefit, and the risks associated with iron overload are great. Supplementation is appropriate for certain populations, including athletes moving from sea level to training at altitude, and especially for individuals diagnosed with IDA and those with chronic low iron intake (vegetarians, athletes in weight-sensitive sports). In the case of the latter group, iron status should be assessed before initiating supplementation. While it is unclear whether individuals with iron deficiency in the absence of anemia or those experiencing iron depletion will see improvements in performance with iron supplementation, it is believed that in this population supplementation should be initiated to prevent the progression to IDA, especially in the presence of symptoms such as fatigue and poor performance (DellaValle 2013).

Iron salts are the most commonly consumed forms of supplements, with ferrous forms having better bioavailability than ferric forms. Ferrous fumarate and gluconate are available, though ferrous sulfate is the most common. Different forms of iron have varying amounts of elemental iron, which references the amount of iron available for intestinal absorption. For example, 100 mg of ferrous sulfate has 20 mg of elemental iron, though the amount of elemental iron in a supplement will be listed on the label making it easy to determine. As with food sources of nonheme iron, coconsumption of vitamin C and consuming meats, poultry, and seafood will improve iron absorption, whereas phytates, calcium, and caffeine can impede absorption. Helping athletes understand these factors and providing practical tips for improving absorption (such as eating an orange when consuming a supplement) will support improvements in iron status. Another consideration is taking a supplement already containing vitamin C that are commercially available.

The amount of iron needed depends upon the degree of deficiency, and iron repletion can take several months. A dose of 100 mg of ferrous sulfate has shown to be effective in increasing serum ferritin levels over 6 to 8 weeks, though a higher dose may be warranted with severe

IDA (Goodman et al. 2011). Side effects of iron supplementation may be experienced, including gastrointestinal distress, nausea, and constipation; if these are experienced, the dosage can be lowered. Dividing the dose up into two smaller doses a day can also improve side effects. Once iron levels reflect healthy iron stores, supplementation should cease in order to prevent toxic effects of excessive iron. However, given that individuals who were once diagnosed with iron deficiency are at greater risk for deficiency in the future, these individuals should be encouraged to focus on dietary sources of iron.

Consistent monitoring is recommended to assess iron status and avoid excessive supplementation. Those undergoing a supplementation regime should ideally get their serum ferritin levels checked every 8 to 12 weeks. Individuals at risk for iron deficiency, including those with a history of IDA, vegetarians, individuals with bleeding or menstrual disorders or both, and those with symptoms such as fatigue and poor performance should get assessed periodically.

In summary, female athletes are at greater risk for iron deficiency than their nonathletic and male counterparts, and thus should be screened routinely for iron deficiency. It is evident that performance is impaired with IDA, and while it is less clear if performance suffers with iron deficiency in the absence of anemia, iron supplementation may be warranted given symptomology. A moderate supplementation protocol should be initiated as well as educating the athlete on dietary strategies for increasing iron intake. Athletes undergoing iron supplementation should be monitored to avoid iron overload, and future screenings should continue given they are at increased risk for future deficiency.

Nutrient Needs of the Vegetarian Athlete

A vegetarian approach to food can be a healthful and nutrient-dense way to meet one's nutrient needs. Vegetarian diets have been shown to decrease one's risk for many chronic diseases including heart disease, diabetes, obesity, hypertension, and certain cancers; this is attributed not only to the absence (or reduced presence of) animal products, but also to the increased consumption of fiber, antioxidants, vitamins, minerals, and phytochemicals that can be found in these diets. However, becoming vegetarian does not guarantee these benefits since a vegetarian approach can also include a high consumption of fat, refined flours, and added sugars, depending upon an individual's food selection. While a vegetarian diet (depending upon the type of vegetarianism chosen) can meet all of one's nutrient needs, this dietary approach may result in greater risk for inadequate intakes of certain nutrients. This emphasizes the importance of appropriate nutrition education on meeting nutrient needs as well as the necessity for a well-thought-out dietary plan.

There are a variety of ways in which a vegetarian may approach dietary intake, and Table 8.6 identifies various approaches that may fall under this heading. In addition to more traditional approaches, newer terms such as flexitarians and nutritarians are being used to describe individuals who may include some animal products but, in general, focus on a plant-based diet; in the case of a nutritarian, the emphasis is on selecting high nutrient quality (or nutrient-dense) foods. These terms highlight the benefit of a plant-based dietary approach for anyone and including athletes, and regardless of inclusion of animal products, food selection should focus on foods high in nutritional value.

The concept of a vegetarian athlete is not new, and, in fact, vegetarian athletes have been seen to achieve great athletic status. Carl Lewis, the famous Olympic track and field athlete, is one prime example of a vegan athlete excelling in sport. Of course, given the dietary restrictions of a vegetarian approach, these athletes need to be educated on the importance of nutrient-dense foods and avoiding micronutrient deficiencies. This includes education on which nutrients are at increased risk for inadequate intake, as well as dietary sources providing these key nutrients.

Table 8.6 Different approaches to vegetarianism

Type of vegetarian	Foods consumed or avoided
Vegan	Does not consume any animal products
Lacto-ovo-vegetarian	Eat dairy and eggs; avoid meat
Lacto-vegetarian	Eat dairy; avoids egg and meat
Ovo-vegetarian	Eat eggs; do not eat dairy or meat
Pescatarian	Technically not a vegetarian. Eats fish, but not eat meat or poultry
Flexitarian	Plant-based diet, may occasionally consume meat

The sports nutrition practitioner can help develop practical strategies for incorporating these nutrients into the diet and can include meal planning techniques.

Particular Concerns Among These Athletes

Key nutrients at risk for insufficient intake include vitamin B-12, vitamin D, calcium, iron, zinc, iodine, riboflavin, and omega-3 fatty acids. The degree of dietary restriction—that is, the more foods that are eliminated from the diet—the greater the risk of deficiency. For example, lacto-ovo vegetarians may consume ample amounts of these nutrients, while vegans are at the greatest risk of inadequate intake. Whether or not these athletes require additional supplementation depends upon the degree of adequacy of intake, which can be determined through the dietary assessment.

A special note on iron and protein. The previous section on iron status and athletes highlights the greater risk for iron deficiency among female athletes. Additionally, it is estimated that vegetarians may require up to 1.8 times the amount of iron as those who consume heme sources of iron (that is, from animal products). Therefore, it is particularly important to educate vegan athletes on plant sources of iron; supplementation should not be initiated unless iron status has been assessed and found to be deficient. Similarly with protein, the bioavailability of plant sources of protein is not as high as animal sources *in general*, though certain plant foods such as soy are a high-quality protein source. Due to the lower bioavailability of plant protein sources, vegetarian athletes are recommended to consume approximately 10 percent more protein, or ~1.3 to 1.8 g/kg/day. Many vegetarian athletes do consume this higher amount of protein and it is typically athletes following more restrictive intakes that risk inadequate protein intake.

The sections on calcium, vitamin D, and omega 3 fatty acids can be referenced for other nutrient-specific information. In addition to the micro- and macronutrients that require additional attention, consideration should be paid to overall EI. A high fiber diet that can be seen among vegetarians can also result in reduced EA, particularly due to fiber's effect on feelings of fullness, which can reduce overall EI. Additionally, some individuals use a vegetarian approach as a way to eliminate foods from their diet in efforts to restrict EI. This can be part of a disordered eating pattern and should be explored. In general, it is helpful for the sports nutritionist to ask why an athlete is choosing a vegetarian approach to ascertain if there are unhealthy motivations.

Overall, a vegetarian athlete can achieve optimal health and desired performance goals with this style of eating. The sports nutritionist should conduct a thorough dietary analysis to determine if there are any nutrients at risk for inadequate consumption including specific micro- and macronutrients as well as overall EI. The athlete should be educated on intentional eating practices to meet their nutrient needs, and the practitioner can support the athlete in finding practical strategies for implementing these recommendations.

Definitions

Ketogenic—adjective describing a diet that produces ketones in the body

Menarche—the first menstrual period

Eumenorrhea—regular or normal menstruation

Oligomenorrhea—infrequent menstruation; can be characterized by menstrual cycles lasting longer than 45 days or only having four to nine menstrual cycles a year

Primary amenorrhea—no menarche by age 15

Secondary amenorrhea—absence of three consecutive cycles postmenarche

Sarcopenia—loss of skeletal muscle mass and strength as a result of the aging process.

References

American College of Sports Medicine. 2009. "American College of Sports Medicine Position Stand. Progression Models in Resistance Training for Healthy Adults." *Medicine and Science in Sports and Exercise* 41, no. 3, pp. 687–708. doi:10.1249/MSS.0b013e3181915670

Beals, K.A. 2002. "Eating Behaviors, Nutritional Status, and Menstrual Function in Elite Female Adolescent Volleyball Players." *Journal of the American Dietetic Association* 102, no. 9, pp. 1293–96.

Bratland-Sanda, S., and J. Sundgot-Borgen. 2013. "Eating Disorders in Athletes: Overview of Prevalence, Risk Factors and Recommendations for Prevention and Treatment." *European Journal of Sport Science* 13, no. 5, pp. 499–508. doi:10.1080/17461391.2012.740504

Cogswell, M.E., A.C. Looker, C.M. Pfeiffer, J.D. Cook, D.A. Lacher, J.L. Beard, S.R. Lynch, and L.M. Grummer-Strawn. 2009. "Assessment of Iron Deficiency in US Preschool Children and Nonpregnant Females of Childbearing Age: National Health and Nutrition Examination Survey 2003–2006." *The American Journal of Clinical Nutrition* 89, no. 5, pp. 1334–42. doi:10.3945/ajcn.2008.27151

De Souza, M.J., A. Nattiv, E. Joy, M. Misra, N.I. Williams, R.J. Mallinson, J.C. Gibbs, M. Olmsted, M. Goolsby, G. Matheson, and Panel Expert. 2014. "2014 Female Athlete Triad Coalition Consensus Statement on Treatment and Return to Play of the Female Athlete Triad: 1st International Conference Held in San Francisco, California, May 2012 and 2nd International Conference held in Indianapolis, Indiana, May 2013." *British Journal of Sports Medicine* 48, no. 4, p. 289. doi:10.1136/bjsports-2013-093218

DellaValle, D.M. 2013. "Iron Supplementation for Female Athletes: Effects on Iron Status and Performance Outcomes." *Current Sports Medicine Reports* 12, no. 4, pp. 234–39. doi:10.1249/JSR.0b013e31829a6f6b

Economos, C.D., S.S. Bortz, and M.E. Nelson. 1993. "Nutritional Practices of Elite Athletes. Practical Recommendations." *Sports Medicine* 16, no. 6, pp. 381–99.

Garthe, I., T. Raastad, P.E. Refsnes, and J. Sundgot-Borgen. 2013. "Effect of Nutritional Intervention on Body Composition and Performance in Elite Athletes." *European Journal of Sport Science* 13, no. 3, pp. 295–303. doi:10.1080/17461391.2011.643923

Ginde, A.A., M.C. Liu, and C.A. Camargo, Jr. 2009. "Demographic Differences and Trends of Vitamin D Insufficiency in the US Population, 1988–2004." *Archives of Internal Medicine* 169, no. 6, pp. 626–32. doi:10.1001/archinternmed.2008.604

Girgis, C.M., R.J. Clifton-Bligh, M.W. Hamrick, M.F. Holick, and J.E. Gunton. 2013. "The Roles of Vitamin D in Skeletal Muscle: Form, Function, and Metabolism." *Endocrine Reviews* 34, no. 1, pp. 33–83. doi:10.1210/er.2012-1012

Goodman, C., P. Peeling, M.K. Ranchordas, L.M. Burke, S.J. Stear, and L.M. Castell. 2011. "A to Z of Nutritional Supplements: Dietary Supplements, Sports Nutrition Foods and Ergogenic Aids for Health and Performance–Part 21." *British Journal of Sports Medicine* 45, no. 8, pp. 677–79. doi:10.1136/bjsports-2011-090102

Gropper, S.S., L.M. Sorrels, and D. Blessing. 2003. "Copper Status of Collegiate Female Athletes Involved in Different Sports." *International Journal of Sport Nutrition and Exercise Metabolism* 13, no. 3, pp. 343–57.

Manore, M.M. 2013. "Weight Management in the Performance Athlete." *Nestle Nutrition Institute Workshop Series* 75, pp. 123–33. doi:10.1159/000345831

Mountjoy, M., J. Sundgot-Borgen, L. Burke, S. Carter, N. Constantini, C. Lebrun, N. Meyer, R. Sherman, K. Steffen, R. Budgett, and A. Ljungqvist. 2014. "The IOC Consensus Statement: Beyond the Female Athlete Triad–Relative Energy Deficiency in Sport (RED-S)." *British Journal of Sports Medicine* 48, no. 7, pp. 491–97. doi:10.1136/bjsports-2014-093502

Nichols, J.F., M.J. Rauh, M.T. Barrack, H.S. Barkai, and Y. Pernick. 2007. "Disordered Eating and Menstrual Irregularity in High School Athletes in Lean-Build and Nonlean-Build Sports." *International Journal of Sport Nutrition and Exercise Metabolism* 17, no. 4, pp. 364–77.

Ogan, D., and K. Pritchett. 2013. "Vitamin D and the Athlete: Risks, Recommendations, and Benefits." *Nutrients* 5, no. 6, pp. 1856–68. doi:10.3390/nu5061856

Phillips, S.M. 2014. "A Brief review of Higher Dietary Protein Diets in Weight Loss: A Focus on Athletes." *Sports Medicine* 44, Suppl 2, pp. S149–53. doi:10.1007/s40279-014-0254-y

Rizzoli, R. 2014. "Nutritional Aspects of Bone Health." *Best Practice & Research Clinical Endocrinology & Metabolism* 28, no. 6, pp. 795–808. doi:10.1016/j.beem.2014.08.003

Rolls, B.J., A. Drewnowski, and J.H. Ledikwe. 2005. "Changing the Energy Density of the Diet as a Strategy for Weight Management." *Journal of the American Dietetic Association* 105, no. 5, Suppl 1, pp. S98–103. doi:10.1016/j.jada.2005.02.033

Schoene, R.B., P. Escourrou, H.T. Robertson, K.L. Nilson, J.R. Parsons, and N.J. Smith. 1983. "Iron Repletion Decreases Maximal Exercise Lactate Concentrations in Female Athletes with Minimal Iron-Deficiency Anemia." *The Journal of Laboratory and Clinical Medicine* 102, no. 2, pp. 306–12.

Skarderud, F., T. Fladvad, H. Holmlund, I. Garthe, and L. Engebretsen. 2012. "The Malnourished Athlete–Guidelines for Interventions." *Tidsskrift Norske Laegeforening* 132, no. 17, p. 1944. doi:10.4045/tidsskr.12.0574

Sundgot-Borgen, J. 1994. "Risk and Trigger Factors for the Development of Eating Disorders in Female Elite Athletes." *Medicine and Science in Sports and Exercise* 26, no. 4, pp. 414–19.

Sundgot-Borgen, J., and I. Garthe. 2011. "Elite Athletes in Aesthetic and Olympic Weight-Class Sports and the Challenge of Body Weight and Body Compositions." *Journal of Sports Sciences* 29, Suppl 1, pp. S101–14. doi:10.1080/02640414.2011.565783

Sundgot-Borgen, J., N.L. Meyer, T.G. Lohman, T.R. Ackland, R.J. Maughan, A.D. Stewart, and W. Muller. 2013. "How to Minimise the Health Risks to Athletes Who Compete in Weight-Sensitive Sports Review and Position Statement on Behalf of the Ad Hoc Research Working Group on Body Composition, Health and Performance, Under the Auspices of the IOC Medical Commission." *British Journal of Sports Medicine* 47, no. 16, pp. 1012–22. doi:10.1136/bjsports-2013-092966

Swinburn, B., and E. Ravussin. 1993. "Energy Balance or Fat Balance?" *The American Journal of Clinical Nutrition* 57, no. 5, pp. 766S–70S; discussion 770S–71S.

Torstveit, M.K., and J. Sundgot-Borgen. 2005. "The Female Athlete Triad Exists in Both Elite Athletes and Controls." *Medicine and Science in Sports and Exercise* 37, no. 9, pp. 1449–59.

Whiting, S.J., and W.A. Barabash. 2006. "Dietary Reference Intakes for the Micronutrients: Considerations for Physical Activity." *Applied Physiology, Nutrition, and Metabolism* 31, no. 1, pp. 80–5. doi:10.1139/h05-021

Glossary

- **Certified Specialist in Sports Dietetics (CSSD)**—a Registered Dietitian nutritionist who is an expert in the application of sports nutrition. These individuals have successfully completed the board exam following two years working as a Registered Dietitian with a minimum of 1,500 hours of sports nutrition practice.
- **Energy**—the capacity to do work
- **Joule**—the SI unit of energy or work; equals the energy that is transferred when applying a force of one newton through a distance of one meter
- **Resting energy expenditure (REE)**—equivalent to resting metabolic rate (RMR); the amount of energy needed by the body at rest. Testing conditions are less stringent than basal energy expenditure (BEE), which can result in a slightly higher value than BEE.
- **Basal energy expenditure (BEE)**—equivalent to basal metabolic rate (BMR); the amount of energy needed by the body at complete rest. To be accurate, this must be measured in a postabsorptive state (the individual must not be actively digesting food and should be fasted more than 8 hours) and should be assessed immediately upon waking and before rising in the morning.
- **Adaptive thermogenesis**—the decrease in energy expenditure beyond what could be predicted from body weight or its components as a result of a decrease in energy intake
- **Phosphagen system**—provides an immediate and limited supply of ATP by donating high-energy phosphate compounds.
- **Glycolysis**—the metabolic pathway using glucose to produce pyruvate and energy through the replenishment of ATP.

- **Mitochondrial respiration**—a series of catabolic reactions transpiring in the mitochondria of the cell, requiring oxygen, with the result of producing large amounts of ATP to be used for energy production.
- **Redox reactions**—a chemical reaction where the transfer of electrons between substances results in a change in the oxidation state of atoms.
- **VO_2 max**—the maximum volume of oxygen that can be taken in during one minute of exhaustive exercise; often used as a measure of aerobic capacity.
- **Ergogenic**—performance enhancing. An ergogenic aid is an external influence enhancing athletic performance, and may include performance-enhancing drugs, dietary supplements, and physiological, mechanical, and psychological aids.
- **Glycogenesis**—the process of adding glucose molecules to glycogen for storage in the liver or in muscle cells, commonly stimulated by insulin.
- **Muscle cell hypertrophy**—an increase in muscle cell size.
- **Hyperaminoacidemia**—having excess amino acids in the blood.
- **Gluconeogenesis**—the production of glucose from noncarbohydrates carbon sources including pyruvate, lactate, glycerol, and glucogenic amino acids.
- **Euhydration**—normal state of body water content.
- **Diuresis**—increased urine production
- **Periodization**—the systematic planning of physical training; this involves dividing up the training program into specific phases that each have their own training goals.
- **Macrocycle**—typically a year-long training program with the aim of the athlete "peaking" at the time of major competition. This may include the preparation phase that comprises the bulk of the training volume; the competition phase; and the transition phase, or the off-season period.
- **Mesocycle**—a defined training period, anywhere from two to six weeks, within a macrocycle that has specific training adaptations that fit within the overall training plan. The Mesocycle

can be used to time training volume and intensity to allow the athlete to peak at competition.

- **Microcycle**—characterizes the training program within a short period, typically a week, and includes the number of workouts within this time frame. This may include light days and hard days and has the aim of realizing acute adaptations to training goals. The microcycle goals depend upon where the athlete is within the macrocycle.
- **Nutrient density**—the nutrient content of a food in proportion to the calories it contains.
- **Ergogenic aids**—a physical, mechanical, nutritional, psychological, or pharmacological technique or substance that has the potential to enhance performance
- **Ketogenic**—adjective describing a diet that produces ketones in the body
- **Menarche**—the first menstrual period
- **Eumenorrhea**—regular or normal menstruation
- **Oligomenorrhea**—infrequent menstruation; can be characterized by menstrual cycles lasting longer than 45 days or only having 4 to 9 menstrual cycles a year
- **Primary amenorrhea**—no menarche by age 15
- **Secondary amenorrhea**—absence of three consecutive cycles postmenarche
- **Sarcopenia**—loss of skeletal muscle mass and strength as a result of the aging process.

Industry, government, and academic resources for further inquiry:

- Sports, Cardiovascular, and Wellness Nutrition practice group of the Academcy of Nutrition and Dietetics: www.scandpg.org

Index

OTHER TITLES IN OUR NUTRITION AND DIETETICS PRACTICE COLLECTION

Nutrition Support
by Brenda O'Day

*Diet and Disease: Nutrition for Heart Disease,
Diabetes, and Metabolic Stress*
by Katie Ferraro

*Diet and Disease: Nutrition for Gastrointestinal, Musculoskeletal,
Hepatobiliary, Pancreatic, and Kidney Diseases*
by Katie Ferraro

Weight Management and Obesity
by Courtney Winston Paolicelli

Dietary Supplements
by B. Bryan Haycock and Amy A. Sunderman

Introduction to Dietetic Practice
by Katie Ferraro

Momentum Press is one of the leading book publishers in the field of engineering, mathematics, health, and applied sciences. Momentum Press offers over 30 collections, including Aerospace, Biomedical, Civil, Environmental, Nanomaterials, Geotechnical, and many others.

Momentum Press is actively seeking collection editors as well as authors. For more information about becoming an MP author or collection editor, please visit http://www.momentumpress.net/contact

Announcing Digital Content Crafted by Librarians

Momentum Press offers digital content as authoritative treatments of advanced engineering topics by leaders in their field. Hosted on ebrary, MP provides practitioners, researchers, faculty, and students in engineering, science, and industry with innovative electronic content in sensors and controls engineering, advanced energy engineering, manufacturing, and materials science.

Momentum Press offers library-friendly terms:

- perpetual access for a one-time fee
- no subscriptions or access fees required
- unlimited concurrent usage permitted
- downloadable PDFs provided
- free MARC records included
- free trials

The **Momentum Press** digital library is very affordable, with no obligation to buy in future years.

For more information, please visit **www.momentumpress.net/library** or to set up a trial in the US, please contact **mpsales@globalepress.com**.

www.ingramcontent.com/pod-product-compliance
Lightning Source LLC
Chambersburg PA
CBHW070408270326
41926CB00014B/2757